The Unmasking of Medicine

The Unmasking of Medicine

IAN KENNEDY

London
GEORGE ALLEN & UNWIN
Boston   Sydney

First published in 1981

GEORGE ALLEN & UNWIN LTD
40 Museum Street, London WC1A 1LU

©Ian Kennedy, 1981

British Library Cataloguing in Publication Data

Kennedy, Ian
   The unmasking of medicine.
   1. Medical ethics
   I. Title
   174'.2   R724

   ISBN 0-04-610016-4

Typeset in 11 on 13 point Bembo by Alan Sutton, Gloucester
and printed and bound in Great Britain by
William Clowes (Beccles) Limited, Beccles and London.

Preface

This book is an extended version of my 1980 Reith Lectures, entitled "Unmasking Medicine". Obviously the constraints of six half-hour lectures meant that I could not consider some points either at all or in much detail. So I have taken the opportunity to put a bit more flesh on the bones of my arguments and to add an extra chapter. I have also prepared a fairly extensive bibliography of sources, so as to help the reader whose appetite is whetted to find his way to other materials. This bibliography will also show how wide is the range of materials which someone venturing into this area of study needs to cover.

Perhaps I ought to identify the area. Fundamentally, it is the study of the practice of medicine today. In the United States the area goes by the name of "Bioethics", a word I have never found terribly appealing. Here in the United Kingdom we do not seem to have a single label for it. Ethics and law together with sprinklings of philosophy, sociology and politics are all involved as they relate to medicine.

This is not a field in which it is necessary to be trained in medicine. Indeed, it could be said that it is only someone who is free from any claims which medical professional loyalty may make on his objectivity who can successfully examine the institution of medicine. I am a lawyer and have specialised in the field of medical law and ethics for some dozen years. Of course, a lawyer writing on medicine is, to some doctors, like a red rag to a bull. "What about lawyers? Why don't you criticise them?" are questions I have frequently encountered. My only reply is that I happen to be interested in medicine. This does not mean that I think the legal profession is above examination and criticism, merely that such a task is for someone else.

Obviously, there are some issues, indeed many issues, which have not been dealt with in this book. The ones I have chosen reflect my view of what is important. Others might have made different choices. Furthermore, my choices reflect the need to paint with the broad brush, to explore certain general themes, since this is what I perceive to be the role of the Reith Lectures. It follows that I have tried to resist the temptation to pursue any question or matter in too much detail. This may upset some who look for a detailed treatment of, let us say, abortion, and do not find one. It seems to me that it would have been quite wrong to devote the Reith Lectures to the examination of a few individual topics in detail, although admittedly problems are tumbling over themselves for such consideration. Instead I decided it was appropriate to seek to explore and develop certain more general themes. This book reflects that choice.

Just as with the audience of the Reith Lectures, I would hope that readers will come from all sections of society. I have tried to avoid resort to technical language. It is for me virtually an article of faith that issues of great importance, touching on the way we live, ought to be aired and discussed as widely as possible. It is equally my strong conviction that there is no issue which is too complicated to be discussed before an interested and alert audience, provided it is presented in terms which are readily comprehensible. To argue otherwise is to surrender the power to decide to those who would claim the appropriate expertise, and thus to surrender part of that which is one's citizenship. Of course, it is for others to judge whether I have succeeded in these aims. I can only say that the reception my lectures have so far received has encouraged me to believe that I did reach a wide audience and that, whether they agreed with me or not, the large majority enjoyed the opportunity to explore these issues.

I chose as my title "Unmasking Medicine". My purpose is to ask some questions about the way medicine is thought of and practised, and to offer some ways of responding to what I perceive as problems. Clearly, reference to a mask suggests that a face is being presented which hides the real one. My aim is to expose and then examine the real face of medicine. To change the image, I am suggesting that medicine has developed its myths. My task is to dispel the myths, so as to discover what the truth may be. You will notice that I speak of the real face of medicine. It is the institution of medicine which I am examining. Clearly this means that I must look closely at the role doctors play, since it is around them that much of medicine revolves. Some will take this as just another case of "doctor-bashing", but I hope that on mature reflection they will see my goal as something larger and more worthwhile than that. Indeed, I venture to suggest that, although there is criticism, there is also much that could be of help to doctors, if accepted and acted upon. For one theme I pursue is the need for each person to take greater responsibility for his own life, which includes his health. This can only serve to reduce the burden of responsibility now placed on doctors. I am quite sure we lay people do doctors a disservice by shuffling off on to them a range of problems which they should not be expected to deal with.

I do not intend here to offer some abbreviated version of what I say in the book. But let me offer some signposts. I am concerned with a number of themes. One is that of power – the power of the professional, here the doctor. I contrast with this power the notion of the self-determination of the client, the patient, and his sense of responsibility for himself. Another theme is that of the accountability of the doctor. I argue that there is a need to ensure that the decisions of doctors, to the extent that they are not technical, conform to principles acceptable to all of us. Admittedly, in a pluralist society there may not be any consensus, particularly on such troubling issues as abortion. But this is no reason why, even in such cases, the extent of the range of choices which are tolerable to the society at large should not be identified. Once identified, the doctors should then be expected to operate within them. A further theme is that medicine is, at bottom, a political enterprise.

The choices we make as a society about how we govern ourselves, the values we espouse, dictate the kind of health we have, the kind of medical care we make available. Thus, if we are to improve our health, change our medical care, it is to government, not to doctors, that we must address our arguments. If such factors as poverty, malnutrition, stress, unemployment, and lack of job satisfaction are heavily implicated in undermining our health, it is clear these are not matters which doctors can affect.

Some, particularly the practical among you, will want to know what remedies I suggest, what plan of action I propose. You may well be disappointed that I seem to identify problems, ask questions, but do not offer too many answers. I could reply that it is a task in itself just to seek out the problems and ask the right questions. But I do not rest on this. Instead, my explanation is that I offer a particular view and seek to provoke a debate. If my view is rejected as being inaccurate or otherwise flawed, then so be it. Solutions will not be called for. If, as a consequence of debate, my view or something like it is deemed to be valid, then will be the time for the pursuit of answers, which will grow out of the debate. I offer some leads which may help. I suggest that we aim for a different destination. But I do not dwell greatly on the means of getting there, whether, metaphorically, it should be by train or by car or on foot. I see my role as a catalyst. I suppose I am that most irritating of persons – the one who believes that through discussion and education change for the better will emerge. Call it Utopian if you will. But, if you do, I feel you underestimate the power of ideas.

To some this book will be unpalatable. Certainly, it is aggressive in style and some may say that this is counter-productive in one who hopes to persuade. Well, that is a matter of judgement and I have made mine. I am fully aware that there are doctors who will dismiss (and some already have!) what I have to say as "ludicrous" (*Medical News*, 1 January 1981) or an "outrageous absurdity" (*The*

Lancet, 20 December 1980). This is hardly a surprise. There will always be minds which are closed. Some doctors will feel threatened. That is only natural. Others will say (and some have) that they have heard much of it before. This is, of course, no criticism; since if something is worth saying, it is worth repeating. But they should recall that I am not speaking only, or even primarily, to them. I am seeking to carry the debate out of the hushed halls of Academe into the noisy market-place of ideas. I also like to think, if I may change my metaphor, that, although I have used red and green and yellow and a canvas just like others, the landscape I have painted is not the same as the one painted by the others, either in conception or in detail. I must, at the same time, of course, recognise those writers who have gone before, to whom my debt is great. Illich, McKeown, Muir Gray and Doyal come immediately to mind.

I have no illusions about changing society. I merely add my voice to that of others. Any changes which take place will, and must, come slowly, allowing all of us to adjust. At the same time, I offer this book to provoke some and to stimulate others. I also offer it as encouragement to those who cleave to the values we claim we stand for, a society which respects self-determination, within a context of democratic decision making, and which believes in the pursuit of health and a medical service free at time of use, with equality of access and care.

Let me finally make a couple of points concerning style and organisation. The style throughout is that which I regarded as appropriate for a spoken lecture. I have not changed it. What it lacks in formality is compensated for in its directness. The fact that each lecture was part of a series and yet had to stand alone meant that there was inevitably some overlap of ideas. I have not sought to weed these out. Indeed, in the final additional chapter you will see that I return to several themes already touched upon so as to have the opportunity to consider them more closely. I could, of course, have done so by reworking the original lecture. But,

I decided against this. It seemed to me that it would upset whatever overall structure and balance the lectures have.

It would be wrong of me to end this brief preface without thanking those who have helped me. A Research Fellowship from the British Academy helped me to finance much of my early research. My praise and respect for David Paterson, who produced the lectures for the BBC, cannot be overstated. He is the best of friends. He is a professional, and he is one of the most outstandingly able men I know. The faults in these lectures are mine. Much of the credit is his. George Fischer, Head of the BBC Radio Talks and Documentaries Department, offered me constant support. Peter Leek, my publisher, was suitably patient and a friendly guide. My brothers, Stuart and Alan, tolerated my long conversations and demolished many a bad idea. Andrea Gage looked after me and made it all possible.

IAN KENNEDY

Contents

	page
Preface	vii
1 The rhetoric of medicine	1
2 The new magicians	26
3 Suffer the little children	51
4 "Decisions, decisions . . ."	76
5 The doors of mental illness	99
6 "Let's kill all the lawyers"	116
7 The last taboo	140
Conclusion	167
Bibliography	168
Index	183

1
The rhetoric of medicine

SIX years ago, the American Psychiatric Association took a vote and decided homosexuality was not an illness. So, since 1974 – at least to the A.P.A. – it has not been an illness. How extraordinary, you may think, to decide what illness is by taking a vote. What exactly is going on here?

I have set as my task the unmasking of medicine. It is not that I think there is something sinister behind the mask. But I do detect a sense of curiosity, of concern if not disquiet. The practice of medicine has changed. There is a feeling abroad that all may not be well. This feeling grows out of a sense of distance, out of a sense that medicine is in the hands of experts and sets its own path. *We* can take it or leave it. Heart transplants, the definition of death, the treatment of the dying, the sad fate of Karen Quinlan, the selective treatment of handicapped newly-born babies, the treatment of the mentally ill – there is a long list of issues which are deeply troubling but which seem effectively to be kept under wraps. One of the most successful ways of doing this is by making the issues and problems appear to be medical, technical ones, not really for the rest of us at all. This can be accomplished by the simple device of translating the issue into medical language. I do not mean by this translating it into the technical terms we associate with medicine, but embracing it within the conceptual framework of medicine. The first step on the way to *understanding* modern medicine, looking behind the mask, is to unravel the *rhetoric* of medicine.

Let me begin with the word "illness". It is, you say, a word you understand. You know what it means and it will take more than one curious example from the activities of the American Psychiatric Association to persuade you otherwise. "Illness", you insist, is a technical term, a term of scientific exactitude. Whether someone has an illness, is ill, is a matter of objective fact.

But homosexuality is as much a part of social life after 1974 as it was before. The objective facts have not changed. What has changed is how the particular doctors choose to judge it. This suggests the strangely disquieting insight that illness involves not merely the existence of certain facts. It involves a judgement on those facts. And it is doctors who do the judging. A choice exists whether to categorise particular circumstances as amounting to an illness. Power is vested in the doctor, and the power is not insignificant.

It becomes important, then, to discover whether there are boundaries to this word, this concept "illness". Can it be applied willy-nilly, on the say-so of the doctor, or are there limits to his power? To analyse the word "illness" is to explore the role of the doctor in modern medicine. It is to discover that medical practice is above all a political enterprise, one in which judgements about the proper order and governance of society are made.

But, you ask, are there not *many* conditions about which we would all agree that they constitute illnesses. Of course, the answer is yes, there are. Obviously we all agree that someone with an inflamed appendix is ill, as is someone who cannot breathe very well, even when resting. Equally, we agree that someone with, say, leprosy or cancer is ill. Why do we all agree? It is obvious, you say. Someone with an inflamed appendix *is* ill. He has got appendicitis. But this is a circular argument. We have to go more carefully. What we have is certain facts about the physical condition of a person. We all agree that these are illnesses because we accept two propositions. The first is that there is a normal state in which the appendix is not inflamed and breathing is easy while resting. Second, it is appropriate to judge someone who deviates from this norm as ill. Only if we examine both of these will we understand what is involved in the meaning of the word "illness".

Take the first of the two propositions, that there must be a deviation from the normal state. This seems simple enough. It is not, of course. For a start, it is our convention to call such deviations from the norm illnesses. But let it be clear that there is no logical necessity to call a set of physical symptoms an illness. Others, in other cultures, may view such conditions entirely differently. They may see them as visitations from the gods, as punishments deserved and to be accepted, or as possession by spirits. We cleave to science and the scientific principle of a demonstrable state of normality and a causative agent which brings about an abnormality. Few would object to this convention. Even so, we still have a problem. What is the state we should regard as normal?

A common method of answering this is to have recourse to an analogy drawn from engineering. We think in terms of a machine which has a design, which is the norm, and which malfunctions when it does not perform according to the design. Indeed, in common speech we may describe our car as sick, or ill, or on its last legs. And, by and large, this analogy serves us well. But it has its shortcomings. One weakness is that it is crude. We like to think of ourselves as more than machines. We have emotions, moods and feelings which affect profoundly our physical state. A further weakness is that we may not all agree on the design, the blueprint, against which to measure our performance or our state. For example, women have the capacity to bear children. In the old days, it was considered part of the design for women that they bore children. A woman who did not bear children departed from this design. She was to that extent abnormal. She was described as barren, a term with connotations of illness as well as some notion of moral judgement upon her. You will recall that Julius Caesar urged his wife to touch Antony so as to be cured of her barrenness. To some extent we have changed our view of the design for women. There is probably less inclination now to attach to childless women a term suggesting illness or moral judgement.

The point is clear. What is the normal state against which to measure abnormality is a product of social and cultural values and expectations. It is not some static, objectively identifiable fact. As views and values change, so the norm will change. So, if illness has as its first criterion some deviation from the norm, some abnormality, it too will vary and change in its meaning.

Furthermore, I suggested a moment ago that there is a relationship between calling someone ill and making a moral judgement about him. The same abnormality can at different times be illness or evil. When we describe someone as ill we often say that he has got something wrong with him and the word "wrong" can also imply lack of moral worth. Before the days of modern medicine it was common to regard conditions we now regard as illnesses as being attributable to possession by evil spirits. For example, some of those accused of witchcraft by Cotton Mather in seventeenth-century Massachussetts would probably now be described as epileptics or suffering from Huntington's chorea, a fatal congenital illness characterised by uncontrollable shaking and gradual mental degeneration. They would be seen as ill, and certainly not as evil.

On the other hand, we have fluctuated in our views as to whether the user of certain drugs or the alcoholic is ill or evil. The user of morphine and later heroin was regarded in the late nineteenth century as someone perhaps deserving of sympathy because of his dependence on "medication". He was, however, still someone worthy of respect or a position of authority. Estimates suggest that between 2 and 3 per cent of the U.S. population were habituated and dependent upon opiates at the end of the nineteenth century. Such a proportion in the U.S.A. now would be about eight times the number of present-day users of heroin. Within twenty years the users of opiates could be divided into the ill and the evil. Troy Duster, in his book *The Legislation of Morality*, cites an article by G. Swaine in 1918 in the *American Journal of Clinical Medicine* in which users were divided into two classses.

"In class one", Swaine wrote, "we can include all of the physical, mental and moral defectives, the tramps, hoboes, idlers, loaders, irresponsibles, criminals and denizens of the underworld . . . In these cases, morphine addiction is a vice, as well as a disorder resulting from narcotic poisoning. These are the 'drug fiends'. In class two, we have many types of good citizens who have become addicted to the use of the drug innocently and who are in every sense of the word, 'victims'. Morphine is no respecter of persons, and the victims are doctors, lawyers, ministers, artists, actors, judges, congress-men, senators, priests, authors, women, girls, all of whom realise their condition and want to be cured. In these cases, morphine-addiction is not a vice, but an incubus, and, when they are cured, they stay cured."

What had happened was that in 1914 the Harrison Narcotic Act had been passed. A crucial provision was that a user could obtain his heroin or morphine only on a doctor's prescription. In 1919 the U.S. Supreme Court, in *Webb* v. *U.S.*, considered what was the effect of the pro-vision in the Act that a prescription could be given only for "legitimate medical purposes". The Court decided that "a prescription of drugs for an addict, not in the course of professional treatment in the attempted cure of the habit, but being issued for the purpose of providing the user with morphine sufficient to keep him comfortable by maintaining his customary use was not a prescription in the meaning of the law and was not included within the exemption for the doctor–patient relationship".

The habituated user, cut off from a lawful supply, had to go underground, to the criminal black market. The climate was created for what Duster calls "a moral reassessment of what had previously been regarded as a physiological problem". Opiate users could be reclassified as criminals and therefore morally evil. The motive for the Harrison Act was well-meaning paternalism, to protect an unsuspecting population from the habituating qualities of opiates. The result was to allow drug use to be seen in moral terms.

There is, in many contexts, a subtle relation between ill and evil whereby the description "ill" can carry with it a marked undertone of moral judgement and condemnation. For example, an illness often takes on a metaphorical quality whereby it becomes a condemnation of some social ill. Something is a cancer in our midst or is pestilential. Or a person may be said to be ill – as is, for example, the alcoholic – but in the next breath it may be said that he has only got himself to blame, or he is very weak, where weak is synonymous with lack of moral strength. Running through all these examples is, of course, the central theme of responsibility. As our views of each person's power to exercise dominion over his life change, so will our concept of the borders between illness and evil. Evil is deemed to be a product of a person's choice and therefore something for which he is responsible. Illness, by contrast, is something which overtakes him. Once ill, he is absolved from the ordinary responsibilities of everyday life.

Turning now to the notion of possession, this too has retained some vitality. The old notion of illness being caused by devils or demons possessing the sufferer fell before the onslaught of scientific medicine. But scientific medicine has not abandoned the notion of possession. Indeed, it is as strong as ever. What has changed is the identification of the possessing force. Demons become germs, spirits become diseases.

So illness, a central concept of medicine, is not a matter of objective scientific fact. Instead, it is a term used to describe deviation from a notional norm. So, a choice exists whether to call someone ill. The choice depends upon the norm chosen and this is a matter of social and political judgement. As the great American scholar Oliver Wendell Holmes remarked, at the end of the nineteenth century, "the truth is that medicine, professedly founded on observation, is as sensitive to outside influences, political, religious, philosophical, imaginative, as is the barometer to the changes of atmospheric density". Ordinarily there will be widespread agreement about what objective facts, what physical states are appropriately described as abnormal. But this does not belie the fact that there is an inherent vagueness in the term "illness". And this is only the beginning. Even when it has been decided that the physical conditions warrant the description "abnormal", there is still the second step. They have to be *judged* to be an illness. An evaluation has to take place.

This should cause us to pause. Who does the evaluating? What are the values involved? Does this mean that the vagueness we previously noticed is compounded? Does this mean that the concept of illness can be manipulated, that it has no clear and certain boundaries? We began with the cosy assumption that illness was a descriptive term, applied to a set of objective facts. It appears now that illness is an indeterminate concept, the product of social, political and moral values, which, as we have seen, fluctuate. The implications of this will strike you immediately. If illness is a judgement, the practice of medicine can be understood in terms of power. He who make the judgement wields the power.

Let me explain what follows from this. The treatment of illness is for doctors. A social institution has grown up defined and managed by doctors, the role of which is to persuade us that our preoccupations must be related to them, and them alone (since they alone have competence).

We appear, perforce, naked both physically and emotionally. However willing we may be, and however well
intentioned the doctor, it is hard to overstate the power
which this vests in the doctor. It is hard to overstate how
such a social arrangement may undermine the notion of
individual responsibility and of course, ultimately,
individual liberty.

Michel Foucault, a contemporary French philosopher,
captures the point perfectly, as Richard Sennett make clear
in his review in the *New Yorker* of Foucault's most recent
book, *The History of Sexuality*. Foucault, writes Sennett,
argues that "in the modern world all too often there is no
clear line between concern for the welfare of others and
coercive control of their lives". "A new kind of power
relationship has arisen in modern society," he goes on.
"Authorities who understand our bodies have gained the
right to make and enforce rules about morality." The nature
of the power relationship is seen in terms of confession,
now to medical rather than priestly "authorities". In the
past the person who confessed furnished the raw data, the
confessor the meaning, and so it is today, according to
Foucault.

Interpretation and with it judgement and prescription
become the preserve of authority, since, knowing what we
do not know about ourselves, doctors acquire the right to
show us how to behave. Let me take this further. So far, I
have mentioned only the interplay between illness and
morality. A far more significant interplay exists on a
political and social plane. Just because illness is associated
with objective facts, it appears that illness *is* those facts, that
illness is a thing. But, as we have seen, illness is not a thing,
it is a judgemental term. Being ill is not a state, it is a status,
to be granted or withheld by those who have the power to
do so. Status connotes a particular position in society,
assumed only after satisfying others that certain conditions
have been observed.

Let me explain. Consider Mr Smith. He works on an

assembly line. He finds the work dull and tedious. One day, he decides he has had enough and would like just a few days at home. He presents himself to his doctor and asks for a sick note, excusing him from work. Let us analyse this process carefully. The first stage is the understanding by Smith that he needs authoritative affirmation that he is ill. He may decide he is ill, indeed it is a feature of modern medicine that, outside emergencies, it is the individual that makes the first decision concerning illness. He stakes a claim to illness. But his decision is not enough. The monopoly power to confirm or deny the presence of illness rests with the doctor. Notice I used the word power, not skill, since it is more than a technical skill. It is, as I have already said, a social and political power. The doctor may say, "Yes, Mr Smith, you ought to have a few days off", and then add a diagnostic tag such as stress or overwork (overwork being clearly an evaluative term). Smith then gets his sick note. Or the doctor may say, "There is nothing the matter with you, Smith." His notes may read, "Another malingerer".

What process is involved here? What sort of term is "malingering"? It involves a judgement that Smith ought to be working and that the doctor is not going to aid him in avoiding this responsibility. Another doctor could just as well decide otherwise. Besides the power the doctor has to manipulate the concept of illness according to his (the doctor's) or the general population's view of what is socially or politically proper, several other points emerge from this example. One is that a major use of the term "illness" is in a functional sense. Is the person able to function in the role he has? Consider the power this gives the doctor. He may have no idea of what life on an assembly line is like, yet he has the power to decide whether Smith should get back to it or not.

Second, it suggests that the function most clearly involved in the notion of illness is the capacity to work, at least as regards adult males. Health comes to be defined as the ability to work. Of course, this is no new thing. The great public health reforms of the nineteenth century were motivated more by economic than humanitarian considerations. As Henry Chadwick wrote, "Of all those who are born of labouring classes in Manchester more than 57 per cent die before they attain 5 years of age, that is, before they can be engaged in factory labour."

Third, it follows from this that Smith the complainer is not seen as a unique individual with unique needs but rather as a unit in an economic system. The doctor reflects and enforces the values of the day. Productivity is expected of labour. Rest is a reward to be earned.

Fourth, there exists always the opportunity to exercise class bias in the ascription of illness. The blue-collar worker may be conceived of in terms which demand that, whether through brutishness or fortitude, he be less susceptible to stress while the white-collar worker is deemed, probably quite wrongly, to be exposed to greater stress and to warrant more sympathy and tolerance. After all, he works with his brain – an argument which ignores the proposition that mindless work may by its very mindlessness be that much more stressful. There are, of course, numerous other examples of class bias in the manipulation of the concept of illness. For example, consider what happened behind the trenches during the First World War. The private who offered the excuse of shell-shock to explain his wandering off or his refusal to obey orders ran the risk of being shot. The officer was classified LMF, "lacking moral fibre", and was shipped back to Britain. Victorian ladies of the middle class were seen as victims of their bodies, prone to nervous emotions and needing to rest. This view did not, however, extend to those women working long hours in the factories or the mills.

I choose the example of the sickness certificate for Mr Smith not because it suits my purpose but because it is so common and so clear. The conclusion exists that illness is a spurious scientific term and that the doctor in purporting to determine its existence as an objective fact is engaged in a series of moral, social and political choices which we permit him to make. Of course, many doctors find the position they are in most unsavoury. Frequent protests led the Department of Health to change the form of the sickness note in 1976. But the basic system remained and with it the power. The doctor is engaged in a process of socialisation, of ensuring that the prevailing social and political attitudes and values are reinforced and are adhered to by those who, by their behaviour, may be seen as potential deviants. For, as Muir Gray puts it, "deviance is not a property inherent in certain forms of behaviour: it is a property conferred upon these forms by the audience which witnesses them".

If you remain unconvinced of the view I am advancing, consider Mrs Jones. Married at nineteen, she is now thirty-five. She stays at home all day, while her husband is at work and their children are at school. She has grown to dread and despise the tedium of her life. She finds her husband boring. She feels trapped. She has ambivalent emotions towards her children. Life, she feels, is passing her by. She finds herself crying most days. She decides to visit her doctor. She has diagnosed herself as needing help and chosen the doctor in the absence of other obvious candidates as the appropriate provider. She may not think of herself as ill. Indeed, in previous times she may have consulted her priest although not thinking of herself as sinful or in danger of perdition. Her doctor tells her that she is anxious and depressed, something she already knew. The doctor can then confer on her the status of ill, if he so chooses, by offering to treat her through the use of his medical expertise. He will provide antidepressants or tranquillisers. More than two-thirds of all prescriptions for such drugs are for women rather than men. It may be no coincidence that women appear fifteen times more frequently than men in advertisements for mood-changing drugs.

What does this commerce between the two of them signify? The doctor is prepared to use the flexible term "illness" to embrace Mrs Jones's condition. By so doing, he

endows himself with power over her and satisfies his own
and her desire that something be done. A further implication is that he affirms that Mrs Jones is ill, because is not
he treating her? He affirms that her condition is abnormal
and that medical intervention is therefore warranted to bring
her back to normal. Other women cope. Coping is good.
Coping is the norm. But Mrs Jones's complaint is her
dissatisfaction with a social and economic order which robs
her of independence and ties her to her home. The doctor
cannot change the economic and social order, but, with
drugs, he can stop her worrying about it. So that is what he
does. He returns her to the ranks of unhappy women who
no longer feel the pain. By so doing, of course, he prevents
the rancour she feels from being expressed in political or
social terms. The social and economic *status quo* is maintained, through the agency of the doctor. He becomes, once
again, an agent of the prevailing social system ensuring that
its values persist. This is not to say that the doctor's role is
sinister or conspiratorial. In some large part the doctor acts
as a socialiser quite unwittingly. His education has trained
him to see illness and to try to ease pain, even if by so doing
he merely drives the cork deeper into the bottle so making
uncorking that much more explosive.

The doctor is not, of course, wholly innocent, though he
may be disquieted. He knows what he is doing. He must
resort to such arguments as "Should I just let her go on
being unhappy? That would be too cruel." It is a hard
question to decide which course is the more cruel. Recently
a Liverpool doctor, many of whose patients are now
unemployed, described on BBC radio how they came to
him for "a Vali", a Valium tablet. He said he really did not
know what to do. He could not give them a job. They were
clearly anxious and depressed, yet he was reluctant to prescribe drugs for something he saw as a political ill. Of
course, we the public have connived at this exercise of
power by the doctor, out of ignorance, or trust, or – inter-
estingly – even out of choice. We may well seek sometimes

the childlike irresponsibility that illness endows upon us. There is nothing like being ill occasionally. You are waited on hand and foot, excused from responsibility, indulged and pampered. Victorian ladies avoided all sorts of crises by an attack of vapours and a headache has been a godsend to many an embattled female. As Susan Sontag argues in her book *Illness as Metaphor*, nineteenth-century Romantics developed the idea of invalidism as a pretext for leisure and an escape from bourgeois responsibilities. It was "a way of retiring from the world without having to take responsibility for the decision". We have opted for what Illich has called the medicalisation of life, the conversion of social and political ills into illnesses.

Some of you may say that I have given an exaggerated account, that there is a lack of balance here. Well, the examples of Mr Smith and Mrs Jones, so far from being unusual, are among the most common encounters between doctors and patients. Indeed, close to 10 per cent of all prescriptions written by general practitioners are for tranquillisers, antidepressants, or hypnotic drugs, at an annual cost of about one-fifth of the annual expenditure of the N.H.S. on drugs.

If further evidence is called for, consider the following. To demonstrate the evaluative nature of illness, take someone who had difficulty in breathing as a child. He can be told that there is nothing the matter with him that cannot be avoided by a few simple precautions or he can be told that he is ill, that he has asthma. To choose the latter course is to label him and to cause him to think of himself as an invalid for the rest of his life. From someone who cannot run, he becomes someone who should not run. To illustrate the socially determined nature of illness, take, for example, the medicalisation of bereavement. Someone who is grieving is now deemed to be in need of medical care and, perhaps, drugs. Or again, consider a girl who has a bad bite or crooked teeth. She is told that her teeth need to be corrected. Her condition which warrants medical intervention is that she deviates from a socially determined ideal of beauty. Anyone who does not meet this ideal has something wrong with her. Or again, scratchy throats, runny noses, or headaches can be converted into illnesses and the growth of the speciality of allergy treatment has indeed brought this about. Or again, a study in South Wales showed how tiredness was taken for granted as a normal state of everyday life by members of the working class but was likely to be seen as a sign of illness by those in the middle class. Another example may be the growth of certain mass screening procedures. These have sometimes had the unfortunate consequence of persuading people who felt perfectly well beforehand that they are "susceptible", or "at risk", or in a "pre-whatever-it-is state", thereby causing them to think of themselves thereafter as ill, even though nothing is different. Perhaps the supreme example of this epidemic of illness lies in the area of mental illness. I shall consider this at much greater length later. Suffice it to say here that the categories of mental illness seem never to be closed and that candidates for the status "ill" are constantly emerging to fill the categories developed by those whose interest lies in the continuation of this process, those who specialise in mental illness.

Let me now move to a further point. There is within the concept of illness a further element. We tend to confine the use of the word to certain circumstances. We demand of the aspirant to the status "ill" the condition that he be capable of getting better, of recovering from his illness. Illness is regarded as a transient state bounded by optimism. Notice that we tend not to use the term in a number of situations in which there is a clear deviation from the notion of an objective physiological norm. For example, we do not describe those who have lost a limb, or gone blind, or deaf, as ill. We may use the word "invalid" or "disabled" but not "ill". In using these other terms, we reveal once again the close relationship between the language we use and the values of our society. *In*valid has the same root as in*va*lid, like a bad cheque. It does not work, it has no force, it has no worth. The change in pronunciation helps us to hide the harshness of this judgement and its reflection of the values of production and economic worth. Disabled is only slightly less harsh. The person so described is no longer able, he cannot do, and one adds the words, anything or anything much. Again the values of an industrial, production-oriented society emerge.

Take now the terms "chronically ill" and "terminally ill". As regards chronically ill, there is no optimism here, so the adverb "chronically" is used to signal the fact that this is not ordinary illness, but a special status with its own special rules. The same is true of "terminally ill". This term is a product of the modern obsession with death. Clearly, someone who is dying will not recover. Yet our pathetic search for immortality has led us to think of dying as an illness, because, by so categorising it, we hope, perhaps magically, to introduce a note of optimism, a remote possibility of getting better. But rationally we must separate it from the general status of ill, so again we use the qualifying adverb "terminally". Thus, we are true to reason without abandoning irrational hopes! A final example is the term "handicapped". Once again this connotes someone who is less than competitive in the market and thereby again reflects societal views of life as being rooted in economic terms.

Why do I dwell on this? Circumstances have been marked off in which the term "illness" is not "properly" to be used, or is to be used only with qualification. It is no coincidence that these are areas in which the doctor's power to do anything is much limited. The term "illness" has become reserved "properly" for circumstances in which recovery is possible, or, at least, treatment, intervention can be justified. Thus the doctor gratifies himself in his adopted role as healer, a role identified for him in medical school, and retains his status and credibility with the public, by conditioning his power and claim to competence by reference to the chances of success. This is not to say that doctors cannot do much for the chronically ill or disabled. They both can and do. It is only to say that separate categorisation of such people serves as a signal that what can properly be expected of the doctor is different. A further unfortunate consequence of this process is that persons consigned to a status other than ill "properly so-called" may well be less well thought of and certainly less well cared for. Doctors, for the most part, will opt out of devoting themselves to people who offer no obvious reward, no prospect of achieving something by way of cure. This is perhaps one important but overlooked reason why the handicapped, the chronically ill and the disabled are so severely neglected in our society. The terminally ill may be the exception, because, while it is true that most languish in unhappiness buoyed only by the devotion of nurses, the growth of the societal preoccupation with death has persuaded doctors to enter this field as merchants of hope, at least of temporary respite, through surgery, chemotherapy and the like.

In conclusion, I am not saying that we should abandon the use of the word "illness". I am merely urging that we understand what it involves. Since the diagnosis of illness always calls for a judgement, it is right for us all to consider when it is properly to be applied and who should apply it. We should consider what limits may properly be placed by us on the power of doctors to manipulate the concept. I am not suggesting that we take a vote. But we must make it our business to ensure that the judgements arrived at reflect the considered views of all of us. Each diagnosis is an ethical decision.

So far I have concentrated on the term "illness". Let me now consider the concept of health. Health, if it is to have any useful meaning, must refer to more than the mere absence of illness. It must have a positive quality. For example, a man who, for want of anything else to do, lies in bed all day may not have any illness, may in that sense be well, but would not ordinarily be described as leading a healthy life. Health must refer to all those factors which combine to represent man's aspirations and expectations. But, if expressed in this way, once again you see at once that here is no term of nice exactitude. It is in short an evaluative term, redolent with moral, spiritual, political and social overtones and by no means limited to bodily functioning. This is captured in the World Health Organisation's definition of health as "not the mere absence of disease, but total physical, mental and social well-being". This definition, however, so far from serving as a blueprint for planning and policy, whether for governments or doctors, is often held up for ridicule, even by doctors.

"What is the use of this sort of airy-fairy thinking?" the argument goes. "We cannot do anything about these things. We have got enough on our hands dealing with the illness about us. We cannot make people richer or more comfortable or whatever total well-being means."

But let us consider this ridicule for a moment. To embrace a notion of health which calls for positive political action and the creation of appropriate economic and social conditions is to concede that "health" is fundamentally a political term. This most doctors are unwilling to do. They see themselves and want to be seen as scientists, not the political and social agents I have suggested they often are. And to adopt this approach would be to call for some movement away from investing the great part of our resources in attempting to remedy existing illness (a never-ending exercise), towards the principle of preventing, checking or controlling, through social and political action, many of the conditions which give rise to illness. Very many of the people to whom we are readily prepared to ascribe the status "ill" find themselves ill because they are poor, grow up in bad housing, eat poor food, work, if at all, at depressing jobs, and generally exist on the margin of survival. The doctor, because of the way medicine has developed, sees himself as powerless in these matters, except as a voting citizen along with everyone else. And his professional vote goes to retaining a notion of health tied to illness, because here he is all-powerful. The doctor is the entrepreneur of illness. Quite contrary to the view of Sir James Bryce, that "medicine is the only profession that labours incessantly to destroy the reason for its own existence", the opposite is true. We have abdicated to doctors the power to define health, with the result that it is predominantly defined in terms of illness and disease. And as long as it is accepted that health is the exclusive preserve of doctors, something only they have competence in, this state of affairs will continue. It is a matter of balance. The power now is with the professional. Only when it is realised that health is far too important to be left entirely to doctors, that it is a matter for all of us, will conditions be created for the necessary redirection of effort and resources. Only then will any real movement towards health be achieved.

Let me end my examination of the rhetoric of medicine by considering the word "disease". Disease has become a central concept of medicine. It has brought in its wake a number of unfortunate consequences. Doctor Bernard Dixon remarks in an article in the *New Scientist* that although there may be some slow rethinking of this concept it still wields tremendous force, such that "orthodox medicine is strait-jacketed by it".

Let me explain. If illness involves, at least in part, an abnormal condition, then this abnormality is thought of in terms of a disease. Immediately you will notice the danger, at least intellectually, of this approach. We have seen that illness is not a thing, but a judgement. Nonetheless, preoccupation with disease has meant that we have misled ourselves into thinking of illness in essentialist terms, as having a specific essence, of being a thing. Illness becomes the occupation (or possession) of the body by an entity called a disease, caused by some particular agent. You will notice an earlier religious precursor of this approach, the possession of the body by spirits, a view which still prevails in certain parts of the world. There is a further impeccable pedigree in the case of Pandora, sent as a punishment by Zeus, complete with her box, containing as Robert Graves puts it "all the spites that might plague mankind". The great spites or plagues of the previous centuries, which brought illness and death, were infections, such as cholera, TB, diphtheria, typhoid, typhus, smallpox, whooping cough and scarlet fever. TB accounted for 17.6 per cent of all the deaths in the first Report of the Registrar-General in 1839 and the real figure may have been closer to one-third of all deaths. There was little understanding of how these infections operated, what caused them to break out and how to survive them.

The idea that infection could be caused by germs was developed in the late nineteenth century. These infections are memories now, at least in the United Kingdom and other rich industrialised countries. Contrary to popular view, it was not modern medicine which caused them to disappear. Their disappearance, as Professor Thomas McKeown so clearly demonstrates in his book *The Role of Medicine*, was due to three factors: improved housing and sanitation, improved nutrition and improved methods of birth control whereby demands on food and physical resources were reduced. By the time that prophylactic measures were available against them, these infections had in fact all but disappeared as major threats, at least in terms of bringing widespread death or serious disablement. This is not to overlook the enormous value of vaccination and immunisation in ensuring that pockets of infection do not break out from time to time.

There is no doubt that the disappearance of the threat from the major infections has been a magnificent boon. But in terms of the development of modern medicine it has had two unfortunate consequences. The first is that the elimination of the major infections has served as the basic evidence, the star witness if you will, of the triumph of modern medicine over illness. A mythology has emerged with metaphors of battle, triumph, conquest: the patient's defences are threatened, the tumour is bombarded after invading the body. The doctor is categorised as the crusader constantly called upon to wage a holy war upon the enemy called disease, in some way a third party distinct from doctor or patient. And not only is the doctor fighting a war; it is also part of the mythology, based on the elimination of infectious diseases, that he will win. Disease will be vanquished. Life will be sweet. Of course, when examined calmly, the basis of the claim is suspect. Just as infections in the nineteenth century were not conquered by medicine, so much of today's illness seems curiously resistant to medical attention. Nonetheless, it is thought churlish if not downright treasonous to doubt the story or ask too many questions.

The other unfortunate consequence of the elimination of major infections is that it has provided the intellectual basis for the development and refinement of the notion of disease, as it is now understood. What we now think of as disease is some specific entity, which is caused by an attack on or invasion of a part or parts of the body, or by some malfunction of a part, so as to produce circumstances in which someone complains of feeling ill. The idea has grown up of a one-to-one relationship between disease and its causative agent. The idea of specific aetiology grows out of this, although first suggested by Thomas Sydenham in the seventeenth century. From evil spirit to germ to infection to disease entity, we have seen attempts to reify or personify a something which once identified can be dealt with. The impact of scientific thinking has provided the ideal climate for this development. The earlier Hippocratic tradition of concern for the whole person in his environment, which had its practical worth in guaranteeing that Greek colonies were established in healthy places, has been ousted by the post-Renaissance view that illness is a mechanical failure. The Cartesian notion of the body as a machine has remained a central thesis. Like the machine, the body has functioning parts, each of which, with proper taxonomical skill, skill in classifying, has to be listed and its function explained. And, just as the machine will not run for long if a fan-belt breaks or a gear cog is stripped, so your body will not function properly if, for example, your kidneys malfunction or are attacked. Humans have been reduced through the application of impeccable scientific skills to ambulatory assemblages of parts. Just as medical scientists have identified and tagged the parts of the body, they have persuaded themselves that they can identify and tag those things called diseases. We have witnessed a great flowering in taxonomy whereby genus, species and sub-species of disease have been set down.

Two observations are in order. First, intellectually satisfying as it may be to develop this taxonomy, it is of little use unless it leads to being able to do anything. Often medical care begins and ends with diagnosis. Second, and far more serious, disease theory has led to an attitude whereby the malady is seen as somehow separate from the sufferer. The disease is what has to be treated, not the person. But we are more than a set of functioning parts. To regard us as such, as machines, is to overlook the great complexity of each of us. It overlooks the subtle inter-dependence and interrelationship of the parts which make up the whole. For example, in a paper published in the *New England Journal of Medicine* in December 1979, Vaillant reported on a study of the health of 204 men over four decades. He demonstrates clearly that the physical health of the subjects in midlife was significantly related to their state of mental well-being, as illustrated by such indicators as job satisfaction, job promotion, recreation with others, marital stability and holidays.

What is wrong with the concept of disease is not that there is no malfunctioning part. There may be. Rather, it is that medicine has come to concentrate on it to the exclusion of all else. Disease theory has induced a sort of medical tunnel vision. What is not seen, as one critic puts it, is the sick person in all his wholeness and variability. Of course, there are doctors who do try to treat the person rather than just the disease. To them what I am saying may appear unwarranted criticism. I would reply by saying that the mentality of treating the disease is widespread and deeply entrenched. Second, given the estimated average contact time between GP and patient of between five and six minutes, the possibilities for treating the person are slim. In other words, the institutional framework within which medicine is practised militates against such an approach.

Furthermore, it is clearly bad science to conceive of illness in terms of specific diseases caused by specific agents. As René Dubos has pointed out, when Robert Koch announced his discovery of the tubercle bacillus he should have realised that all in the room must have been exposed to it in their lifetime, yet they had not suffered from TB. Thus the bacillus was only part of the story. Nutrition, fatigue and other environmental factors were as important in converting something harmless to some into something deadly to many. In Ecuador, for example, the World Bank reports that measles has a mortality rate 247 times higher than in the United States.

But this alleged scientific approach receives constant reinforcement from two principal sources. First, it is socially and intellectually gratifying for doctors to think of themselves and be thought of as scientists. It connotes working in the realm of knowledge and truth, light years away from the barber and the bleeder of the past. It carries a desirable social cachet. Furthermore, it allows for specialisation and sub-specialisation in tune with the taxonomical categorisation of diseases. This allows doctors to mark themselves off from each other, and by creating the supply they provoke the demand. Diseases follow the categories, not vice versa, and, of course, specialisation carries its own risks for the patient. As one wag has put it, surgery is often like killing a fly on a window-pane with a hammer. You kill the fly, but also smash the window. "But", he went on, "if you have a hammer in your hand, everything starts to look like a nail."

The second source of reinforcement for the notion of

disease comes from those who have a vested interest in the continued vitality of the notion of specific disease entities. I think particularly of the pharmaceutical industry. The relation between the manufacturers of pharmaceutical products and medical education warrants careful attention. In the middle of the nineteenth century it was discovered that by-products of coal and later petroleum refinement could be used to manufacture synthetic dyes, chemicals and drugs. Production of pharmaceutical products grew in conjunction with the development of the petroleum and petrochemical industry. If doctors could be persuaded to reorient medicine towards the notion of pharmacotherapy, then, clearly, here were riches indeed. Enterprises such as the Rockefeller organisation began to pour some of their wealth into educational foundations. The major interest of these foundations was medicine. In 1910, Abraham Flexner, a professional educator, produced in the United States his famous report on medical education commissioned by the Carnegie Foundation. He recommended a shift to science-based, professionalised education which would exclude other approaches to medicine, thereafter stigmatised as quackery. Pharmacology was to be an integral part of the curriculum. The approach to health was to be intervention-ist, including the use, not surprisingly, of drugs. Thereafter medical education was massively funded by foundations whose money came from petrochemical and pharmaceutical products. Rockefeller wealth was the largest single private source of capital for medical science and education. Eli Lilly, the drug company, has spent $250 million on medical schools in the United States over the past fifty years or so. The aim, as the Director of Research of a Congressional Committee put it, was to produce a curriculum designed to indoctrinate the student, particularly in the use of drugs.

An early worker in the field, Paul Erlich, coined the term 'the magic bullet' to describe Salvarsan, the drug which was developed around 1910 to treat syphilis. The metaphor of the bullet is of course intended. The disease existed as a specific entity and would by the application of the drug be eliminated. One unfortunate feature of the metaphor, which is with us more and more now, is, of course, that bullets are only as good as the aim with which they are fired. Furthermore, they tend often to fail to discriminate between the intended target and other things behind, in front, and round about. But the image has been enormously successful, so that modern medicine is now almost totally preoccupied with disease identification and disease-specific response, "symptom-swatting", as one writer has put it. In effect, of course, there are occasions in which recourse to drugs more closely resembles writing the name of your intended victim on a bomb and then throwing it into a crowded restaurant where he is eating. Indeed, the term "side-effect" has had to be coined to designate "unwanted" effects. An effect is an effect for all its being called a side-effect. This is an obvious case of sleight of hand.

This is not to say of course that all pharmacological intervention is misconceived. This would be stupid, in the light of such magnificent developments as the sulphonomides and the antibiotics. It is to say that it has helped to produce or reinforce an attitude to illness which is wrong-headed. First, by concentrating on disease, a form of medicine has developed which, besides being mechanical, is conceived of as a rescue or repair service. You wait metaphorically until the car does not work and then you seek to make it work by squirting oil at it or changing some part. Second, the major infections have gone, largely without the help of medicine, and analogies or analyses based upon them are unhelpful. It seems clear that the traditional response of disease identification and disease-specific intervention has made little impact on the incidence of the present ills we endure, though it may have made some easier to endure. Third, to concentrate on illness in the form of disease-entities diminishes us both spiritually and physically. Illness, feeling ill and wanting assistance, implies a process far more complicated and subtle than the metaphorical replacement of a fan-belt. Finally, it is wrong-headed in that, by thinking of illness in terms of disease, we have been led to believe that diagnosis leads to cure.

This, sadly, is far from accurate. There is little to be gained from labelling if not much can be done once the label has been arrived at. And of course the history of modern medicine in overall terms is that just as it was not responsible for the elimination of infections in the nineteenth and early twentieth centuries so it has had very little impact on the death rate since then. It has had considerable impact on the sickness rate from certain ills, but only limited success in the case of others, particularly those which are the most common amongst us, such as tooth decay, digestive disorder, skeletal and muscular disabilities, the common cold, heart ailments, coughs and bronchitis, accidents at work and home, stress, pain and unhappiness. But the myth persists. The whirligig of disease identification goes round and no one seems anxious to stop it or get off. I do not say we should not use the word "disease". I merely urge that we understand the dangers implicit in its use.

I have examined three of the central concepts of modern medicine. You have seen some of the implications they hold. They imply judgement and evaluations. If we are to take back power to control our lives, we can and must examine these judgements and evaluations. We must notice how they are applied. We must be sure they conform to our sense of what is right or appropriate. We must become the masters of medicine, not its servants. Let there be no misunderstanding: in the politics of medicine, it is we who must have the power, we who must set the policies. Educating ourselves in the language of medicine is the first step. Our next step is to look at the way modern medicine has developed – and examine how in many respects it has taken the wrong road.

2

The new magicians

MY view can be stated briefly. Modern medicine has taken the wrong path. An inappropriate form of medicine has been created, in large part by doctors and medical scientists, and eagerly accepted by a willing populace. I will go further. The nature of modern medicine makes it positively deleterious to the health and well-being of the population. We have all been willing participants in allowing the creation of a myth, because it seems to serve our interests to believe that illness can be vanquished and death postponed until further notice, while it serves the interests of doctors to see themselves and be seen as, if not miracle workers (and of course they would be the first to deny this), then at least possible miracle workers.

Science has destroyed our faith in religion. Reason has challenged our trust in magic. What more appropriate result could there be than the appearance of new magicians and priests wrapped in the cloak of science and reason? Please understand that it is we, all of us, who have hitched our wagon to the wrong star, scientific medicine. The unhappy consequence is that medicine is perceived and pursued in ways which do not best serve the needs of society. We do not put to best use the skills and abilities of those who have become its practitioners.

Let me explain in a series of points what I see as the path

taken by modern medicine and how it may be the wrong one. I intend to concentrate on doctors and their attitudes and training. They may represent only 7 per cent of the National Health Service work-force, as against, for example, nurses, who represent 43 per cent, but it is they, the doctors, who spend money and hold the power. As the Royal Commission on the National Health Service put it: "They are responsible for initiating the expenditure in the National Health Service," and "play an important role in the management of the financial resources of the service." Let me make it clear at the outset that what is involved here is a question of emphasis and balance. I know we can all point to many worthy features of medicine. But on balance I find modern medicine wanting.

First, as now taught and practised, medicine is avowedly and self-consciously scientific. Far be it from me to stand against the tide of history and suggest there is more to understanding and caring than contained within the four corners of science. But an education which demands high skills in scientific subjects before going to medical school, and involves years of breathing the heady air of one field after another of scientific endeavour once there, produces what it is intended to produce: a doctor who sees himself as a scientist. It may not produce what is so often needed: someone who can care. I am not suggesting that medical education should not be scientific. Of course it must. But room must be found for other disciplines, particularly the humanities.

In his survey of medical education in 1978, *Quest for Excellence in Medical Education*, Sir George Pickering complained of the growing regimentation of the doctor in training, whereby the student is forced into an intellectual strait-jacket. Changes intended to cause doctors to address the social context of a patient's complaint and seek to involve the various social services have been made and this is now reflected somewhat in practice. But a fundamental problem remains, in that the doctor still sees himself as separate from these services, to which, at some point, he hands over his patients. As the 1979 Royal Commission on the N.H.S. reported, "Critics of the undergraduate medical curriculum argued to us that medical education was not well-adjusted to the working world, that . . . it produced a doctor whose skills, attitudes and expectations were sometimes poorly related to the health problems and needs of the community."

The late Professor Henry Miller, who was Dean at Newcastle Medical School, wrote, in *Medicine and Society*, that much thought has gone into attempts to reshape medical education away from the old model of basic science followed by the plunge into clinical care. A greater attempt has been made to involve students with patients from the outset and most schools now devote some teaching time to courses which seek to relate medicine to the society in which it is practised. That said, he concluded that the emphasis was still fundamentally scientific, such that the "crisis in medical education still remained unsolved". Pickering concluded that, "for the vast majority of students in Great Britain, the medical curriculum is virtually as it was thirty years ago". Moreover, the science now taught only compounds the problem. It is concerned with reaction, response to ills which already ail the sufferer. Far greater emphasis should be placed on inquiring into the causes and origins of illness, with a view to preventing them. So medicine may be called the healing art, but in the practice of that art it is the scientific method which is portrayed as the best, if not the only way.

My next point is that modern medicine is thought of as dispensing cures. The image created of medicine has increasingly been that of curative science in which the model of the doctor is that of the engineer/mechanic curing a sick engine. This reaches its high point in what I see as an attitude to death in which dying has come to be regarded as an illness. Call it an illness and you hold out hope of treatment, control and even cure. Doctor, patient and family become locked in an unholy *danse macabre*. Medicine provides another variation on the theme of the pursuit of immortality, with the respirator symbolising some kind of Promethean eternity. But the engineer/mechanic model is an unfortunate one. Quite simply, the problems that beset us now do not seem readily amenable to cure. And I speak now of the generality of ills: those that kill us before our time, such as cancer, heart disease, respiratory problems, and accidents; or those that chip away at our daily pursuit of tranquillity – colds and coughs, aches and pains and simple unhappiness. I do not seek, indeed it would be quite wrong, to belittle the contribution scientific medicine has made and continues to make, both in curing infections, at least in their short-term effects, and in controlling and soothing numerous otherwise intolerable conditions – in reducing sickness, even if it has had little effect on mortality.

But, as John Loraine points out in his recent book, *Global Signposts to the 21st Century*, "the enthusiasm for engineering medicine contrasts vividly with the rather meagre advantages which have accrued to health through its application". This is so despite such extravagances as ex-President Nixon's "war on cancer", declared in the National Cancer Act of 1971 and presumably still being fought, although annual deaths from cancer in the United States were up a further 70,000 by 1979. The most common causes of death and the most common debilitating diseases still remain beyond the reach of the doctor. Cures there are not.

The idea of the doctor as an engineer, involved in a curative science, produces a further consequence, which I shall make my third point. It is that doctors are encouraged to adopt the mentality of problem-solvers. Problems exist out there in the world which it is their job to solve. What is wrong with that? Well, it is wrong in several respects. It is a mentality which creates problems. Indeed, the more efficiently doctors look for problems, the more they find and the more problem-solvers we need. It is a mentality which converts modern medical care into crisis care. We wait for a crisis, a problem, then we take it to the doctor and expect him to solve it. It is a mentality which fosters the impression that the problem can be solved, an impression all of us readily adopt. Finally, it is a mentality which ignores the notion that problems can be avoided, that waiting for them to arise and then responding to them is a less than adequate way of providing health care.

Fourth another consequence of perceiving medicine as a scientific exercise has meant that it is conceptualised and practised largely in terms of specific diseases. Medicine is thus committed to a process of reductionism. The totality of a complex human being, the product of innumerable forces, involving subtle balances and interrelationships, is broken down. He becomes no more than a collection of parts, one or more of which is diseased. Each disease then has its particular name, *locus* and nature. It is this entity called the disease which then receives attention, not the person. I am not suggesting that we should abandon the notion of disease. It serves a purpose and anyway it is too much a part of our vocabulary to exorcise it now. But, if illness is seen only in terms of specific diseases, this induces a form of tunnel vision. The very skill of the doctor with detail may cause him to lose sight of the whole. Miss A becomes an X-ray projected on a screen, Baby B becomes a bad case of meningitis, Mr C becomes the pain in the neck at four o'clock. Of course, I readily concede that there are doctors who would regard this as an unwarranted criticism, who seek to practise a type of medicine which looks to all the circumstances of the patient. They are, I would suggest, adopting such an approach despite their formal training rather than as a consequence of it. They are responding to the reality of the problems they confront. Theirs are not as yet, however, the views and values which direct the future shape of medicine.

My fifth point is that modern medicine teaches that the appropriate response of the doctor to our complaint is to do something – something aimed at that disease entity. If he has been educated to think of himself as a scientist problem-solver and if there is a disease lurking somewhere, then it is his job to seek it out and remedy it. This has meant that medical responses have more and more taken the form of action against a disease entity, whether surgical excision, or irradiation, or chemical destruction or, if these are not possible, symptomatic relief. Whatever is decided upon, some form of bodily intervention which is disease-specific is usually sought. Something must be done to satisfy both the expectations of the patient and the professional pride of the doctor, and it has to be done to the disease, which is portrayed in terms redolent of morality or religion as something bad, or wrong, which is possessing the body. The process has become one of applying taxonomical skills so as to identify the disease and then deciding upon the appropriate disease-specific response.

Indeed the process may be even less complicated. One study conducted by members of the Institute of Medical Sociology of the University of Aberdeen has shown that the consultant, knowing the limited range of treatments he has available, is typically concerned from the outset of his contact with the patient with the simple question: "Which treatment is most suitable?" The choice is then validated by appeal to the diagnosis.

What is wrong with this mentality of doing something? It is medicine by reflex: wait for the problem and do something. It causes larger and more important questions to be ignored, such as how the state of affairs came about, or what the long- or short-term effects of the chosen response will be. It is particularly unlikely that the question "Should anything be done at all?" will be raised. These questions will tend to be lost in the display of pseudo-scientific wizardry.

The doctor is not alone in cultivating this mentality. You only have to look at advertisements in the press or on television to see how the notion of disease and disease-specific response is manipulated by drug companies so as to sell their products. Diagrams, effective for all their banality, show target areas with the product winging its way to knock out pain, indigestion, headache or whatever, and of course no one encourages this more than we ourselves. It is so much more satisfying to know that you have arthritis than to be unsure what is the matter. The knowledge operates to put your mind at ease. It could, after all, have been another disease of greater menace on the "Richter" scale. But such knowledge says nothing about whether the illness could have been avoided or what impact it will make on your future lifestyle.

The sixth point concerning the inappropriate form medicine has taken is that medicine is increasingly thought of in terms of hospitals. Indeed, the number of hospitals is often cited as a measure of the quality of health care. For example, as Michael Ryan points out in his book *The Organization of Soviet Medical Care,* the Soviet Union was able to claim in the mid-1970s that, except for Sweden and Norway, it had overtaken all other industrialised nations in the ratio of hospital beds to population size. The implication was that its system of health care had equally advanced, despite the long-standing inadequacy of its primary care services, particularly in the countryside. The nonsense of this approach is obvious. Indeed, apart from units concerned with accidents and, perhaps to a limited extent, obstetrics, the fact that an ever-increasing proportion of our Health Service budget, now 70 per cent, goes to hospitals could be said to be evidence of the failures of health care and how we perceive it.

If ever there was a case of putting the cart before the horse, this is it. If preventive medicine, school health care, community health care and general primary care meant anything, hospitals would be far less needed. Hospitals are the epitome of the problem-solving disease-oriented scientific engineer approach. And this idea of hospital–dominated medicine is constantly reinforced in our minds, if only by such things as radio and television programmes, whether they take the form of a soap–opera or a demonstration of the "gee-whiz" surgical skills displayed recently in the BBC television programmes "Your Life in Their Hands". The reasons are many. Medical students are trained in hospitals. Hospitals are where they learn to see themselves as scientist problem-solvers and curers. Hospitals, particularly teaching hospitals, are where all the interesting problems are. As Miller argues, "there is an excessive concentration on the hospital as opposed to the community, and on the relatively small amount of serious illness that is treated in institutions at the expense of attention to common causes of disablement".

In fact, general practitioners deal with between 90 and 95 per cent of all complaints taken to doctors. Furthermore, a 1973 study, *Present State and Future Needs of General Practice*, published by the Royal College of General Practitioners, showed that the illnesses GPs were consulted about were predominantly minor ones, such as coughs, stomach upsets, tonsillitis and earache. These outnumbered tenfold complaints of major illnesses such as bronchitis and pneumonia. An average GP sees only one or two cases of cancer a year. A congenital abnormality could be expected once in every five years.

Hospital doctors see themselves, and encourage others to see them, as an elite. Those in the teaching hospitals are, of course, a kind of super–elite, leaders of the medical world, shapers of medical education. These teachers become the role models for the future. To borrow Professor Miller's words, "The company of biochemists and geneticists remains more stimulating and more attractive to the bright young medical man than that of social workers and chiropodists." Indeed, since the creation of the National Health Service, the number of hospital doctors has increased by over 100 per cent, as has the number of nurses. Hospital specialisations, techniques to advance self-worth and the appearance of need, now number 47, with 11 new ones having been created in the past ten years. This contrasts sharply with the state of affairs in primary and community care. The number of GPs has increased over the same period by 36 per cent. There are only about 1,000 community physicians to serve the whole of the United Kingdom while a large number of vacancies go unfilled. The school health service is woefully understaffed. There are a mere 46 doctors specialising in occupational health per 1 million workers.

Perhaps the final word on this point should rest with Professor McKeown, whose book *The Role of Medicine* deserves the widest audience. He explains how the restricted nature of the work undertaken by teaching hospitals is a consequence of modern scientific medicine being grafted on to the secular voluntary hospitals of the eighteenth century. "These hospitals limited their work to short-term remediable cases which were of greatest interest to the medical profession . . . Thus they excluded the majority of patients who had to be cared for in separate voluntary hospitals . . . or in public institutions (for the infectious, the mentally ill, and the destitute)." Scientific medicine, McKeown argues, reinforced the element of selectivity, by encouraging the notion that the teaching of skills and techniques, to be practised on a small, carefully selected group of patients, was proper preparation for later medical practice.

The consequence is, McKeown balefully notes, that "Professional interest is increasingly absorbed by methods of investigation and treatment whose complexities seem to challenge the attention of the best minds and whose rewards are assumed to justify it. The acute hospital is likely to become still more selective in its admission policies, and the teaching centre with its concentration of resources and abilities, will be the most exclusive of all. Doctors, nurses, and other health workers would then be trained in an environment which reveals a very limited part of the health task, an environment where prestige, rewards, and professional interest all seem to point in the same direction.

After qualification, understandably, they will seek to continue in the activities which were the focus of their training, and only with the greatest reluctance will they consent to enter the massive neglected areas of health care. The large number of patients, particularly among the congenitally handicapped, the mentally ill and the aged sick . . . will be pushed further into the background, and the division of health services into two worlds will be even sharper than it is today."

It should not come as a surprise that we have exported this same mentality to developing countries. The 1980 World Bank Report points to the emphasis on curative rather than preventive care, to the excessive construction of hospitals, and to the education of doctors which is often not geared to their countries' needs, stressing rare diseases and the use of costly equipment while neglecting local health problems. Two-thirds of the health budget of most developing countries goes to medical education and teaching hospitals.

The limitations of adopting this approach in developing countries are illustrated by a medical school programme in Colombia for the hospital care of premature infants. Survival rates were achieved which compared with those in the United States. But 70 per cent of the infants discharged were dead within three months because of infection, malnutrition and general poverty. United Medical Enterprises, which supplies hospitals and medical equipment to Middle East countries, reported 1979 sales at £20 million and pre-tax profits of £2 million. "Business is brisk," glowed the financial reporter of *The Times*. This company, 70 per cent of which is owned by the state-run National Enterprise Board, also operates in Jordan, Nigeria and the Ivory Coast and has just ventured into Uganda. In each of these countries, the average life expectancy is about fifty years (as opposed to about seventy in the United Kingdom). Nigeria has an infant mortality rate of 163 per thousand (as compared with 16 per thousand in the United Kingdom). Uganda is now witnessing the starvation of its people in the north.

Let me now come to my seventh point. With the increasing emphasis on hospitals as the hub of medical care has come another unfortunate feature of modern medicine: that medicine is and should be an enterprise calling for the use of ever more advanced and complex technology. Christian Barnard filled the massive football stadium in Rio twice when he talked of how he performed the world's first heart transplant, yet the majority of his audience could not afford the simple medicine to rid themselves of their intestinal worms. And, in his own country, Oxfam was giving out measles vaccine to malnourished children whose lives were at risk from infection. Schweitzer, in his hospital in Lambarene, becomes a somewhat ludicrous figure, dissipating his energies, albeit for the most noble of reasons. Pressure on the French Government from someone of his stature could well have produced better results for the health of the people of equatorial Africa than losing himself in a primitive jungle hospital, trying to patch up broken lives.

More and more diagnostic aids, surgical tools and supportive equipment, ever more complex, not to mention drugs, the National Health Service bill for which in 1979 amounted to £740 million, are pressed on doctors. The trend is as predictable as it is regrettable. If you are trained to think of yourself as a scientist problem-solver, raised in an environment of white coats and machinery, where people are constantly being monitored and measured, it is inevitable that you will want the latest machine. Recourse to such technology is deemed entirely proper. And those who manufacture such machinery will ensure that the hospital realises that, without this particular advanced scanner, or whatever, the care being offered may well be thought of as substandard. The combination of the administration's nervousness and the doctor's professional self-image is more than enough to ensure that the machine is categorised as essential, to be obtained as soon as possible.

In case you think the picture I am painting is a caricature, consider the National Health Service's distinction awards, which are given to consultants as supplements to their salary. The three specialities most frequently rewarded are, thoracic surgeons, 73 per cent of whom receive awards, neurosurgeons, 67 per cent of whom get awards and cardiologists, 64 per cent of whom get awards. Consultants in geriatrics and mental health, two areas where the technological model fits poorly, although these two areas are blessed with by far the most patients, receive the fewest awards, only 23 and 25 per cent of them respectively. So government, with the aid of the profession, reinforces this technological approach to medicine which I am seeking to illustrate and criticise.

It is fair to say, however, that evidence is beginning to emerge that some at least are having second thoughts as to whether medicine ought to be riding this roller-coaster of advanced technology, not only because of the enormous financial costs involved but also in view of the cost in human terms. R.L. Himsworth, for instance, writing in 1975 in the book of essays *Specialized Futures*, was moved to remark that "At present the expensive enthusiasm for coronary care units is barely contained by administrative and financial considerations and not at all by the lack of evidence that they have a major effect on the overall mortality." After all, what could be more stressful than to be in such a unit!

Miller makes the same point: "The wiring up of a patient with coronary thrombosis to his elaborate instrumentation is a pleasing exercise in technical virtuosity, but evidence of the superiority of the treatment of cardiac infarction in an intensive coronary unit over its simple management at home is not entirely convincing. In fact, the only clinical trial even hints that the opposite may be the case."

Nowhere is the human cost of advanced technology more evident than when applied to those who are fatally ill and dying. Nowhere is the technological imperative of "if we can do it, we must do it" more inappropriate. Heroic forms of intervention, in which the only hero is the patient, become the order of the day, despite doubts as to whether any benefit which may accrue outweighs the hardship endured.

And a further objection is, of course, that technology represents a short-term solution to what are long-term problems. Indeed, to concentrate attention and resources on a form of medicine which reacts to illness already caused means that less interest is cultivated in seeking to discover the origin and causes of a particular illness, and less effort is available to do so. Such a choice between these two approaches to medical care arose, in effect, in the case of polio. At one stage, a decision had to be made whether further research effort and resources should be concentrated on the development of better iron lungs, on the hypothesis that polio was an inevitable incidence of life, or whether they should be spent on the search for a polio vaccine. Those advocating the second alternative finally, and not without difficulty, won the day, with the result that polio is no longer the scourge it was.

The fact remains, however, that the lure of advanced technology is irresistible to the doctor, serving as both validation and vindication of his training and of his image of himself as really the scientist, problem-solver and curer. It is this same mentality which fuels the search for so-called wonder drugs. Though doctors may well frown at the term, the pursuit goes on regardless. Medical research exerts a spell over governments and foundations and thus over the public. The spell is that something is just around the corner, a breakthrough is imminent. We are all mesmerised and the premise largely goes unquestioned, namely that scientific technological medicine is the proper way.

Recently, on 21 February 1980, even Dr Tony Smith, the much respected medical correspondent of *The Times*, was moved to write of "The battle against breast cancer" under the headline "Is breast cancer next for treatment breakthrough?" Interferon, an agent produced by the body and alleged to have therapeutic properties, is the latest candidate. It would of course be wonderful if it were true, but the record of wonder drugs has not been good since the 1950s.

Something by way of an aside is to inquire why interferon warrants scholarly attention while laetrile, the subject of so much controversy in the United States, is condemned. Laetrile is a vitaminic substance, vitamin B17, derived principally from apricot stones. A large number of States, including California, have laws making its sale unlawful. Some, however, claim it as a valuable aid in the treatment of cancer. The medical establishment and the Federal Government's Food and Drug Administration take another view – that its therapeutic value is unproven, that its ingredients make it potentially dangerous and that a patient may delay or even forgo recourse to other accepted forms of cancer therapy and thus not receive the benefit these could bring. To them it is just a modern form of snake oil.

The difference in response cannot be for lack of proof about laetrile: neither it nor interferon has been tested by traditional methods. Nor can it be merely the toxicity of laetrile. It is no more toxic than other substances commonly used in the chemotherapy of patients with cancer. Can it be that laetrile is associated with the counter-culture parodied as vegetarian, sandal-wearing socialists? Can it be that the medical establishment and drug companies are apprehensive about the call for a patient's freedom to act as he wishes as regards his own illness? After all, an estimated $20,000 million a year are spent in the United States on conventional cancer therapy – surgery, irradiation and drugs. Can it be that doctors see the advocacy of laetrile as a blow to their exclusive power, not only to treat disease but also to control the forms of treatment to be used?

My eighth, and final, point concerning the inappropriateness of the way medicine is perceived concerns the notion of illness. I have already spent some time considering this notion and here will confine myself to two matters.

The first is the extent to which the notion of illness has been expanded. We have seen that at base illness is a socially determined and evaluative term susceptible of manipulation so as to confer or deny the status of "ill" on suitable candidates. The growing categorisation of perceptions and circumstances as illnesses has been a feature of the past decades. Much of this expansion has come through the notion of labelling, through the application of taxonomical skills. It does not follow, of course, that because X can now be divided into Y and Z this necessarily represents any advance in knowledge as to how these come about and what can be done about them.

Nowhere is this more true than in the area of mental illness. Indeed, an argument can be made for the proposition that the categories of mental illness came first, the product of theorising, and only later did there emerge a growing army of people to fill these categories. But the process is not limited to mental illness. The response to many of the problems of old age – which are, in fact, problems of, for example, relative poverty, lack of adequate heating, and social isolation – has been to treat them as separate, quite unrelated illnesses, and thereby to medicalise them. The elderly are seen as ill. The consequence is that resources are directed to the provision of doctors, nurses and hospital beds, rather than to redressing the social ills the elderly encounter. In the process, not only is it probable that more money is ultimately spent than would otherwise be necessary, but also the elderly are denied the opportunity to retain the dignity that illness so easily robs them of.

Another example is the ambivalence shown by medicine towards pregnancy, whether to regard it as a normal state or as having at least some of the attributes of illness. Alan Davis, in his book *Relationships between Doctors and Patients*, cautions against the "evangelical approach" to antenatal care. Doctors, he suggests, feel obliged to justify their tests on the grounds of possible risks and dangers, and then have to spend inordinate lengths of time reassuring pregnant women and persuading them that all is well and that pregnancy is quite natural.

A final example is the resort to mass-screening devices to

discover those "at risk", who will, of course, be suitably apprehensive in the future, particularly if little or nothing can be done once the knowledge is gained. The recent report in the *Daily Telegraph* of 15 September 1979 of Dr d'Souza's work at St Thomas's Hospital Medical School in London has not dampened the enthusiasm for such tests, particularly on the part of those who would profit by them. Dr d'Souza's seven-year study concluded that regular medical examinations to detect disease at an early stage were an expensive and inefficient way of raising standards of health. Not surprisingly, the Director of Research for BUPA, the leading commercial scheme for the provision of medical care in the United Kingdom, was quick to criticise the nature of the research and its results. Only three months earlier, BUPA reported that a survey it had conducted had shown that, on average, 540 electricians were less healthy than business managers who were twelve years older. Although this finding could encourage resort to doctors, it is not immediately clear what the doctors would be able to do about it.

One startling use of screening is that now being used in the U.S.A. by certain chemical companies, as reported in the *New York Times* of 3 February 1980. Workers seeking employment are screened for their susceptibility to various chemical agents. Those categorised as "hypersusceptibles" are "weeded out", even though they are within the normal range of human variations. Critics see this as an improper attempt to divert attention from the dangerous conditions of the workplace by blaming the ills that the worker is exposed to on his genes. They point to Aldous Huxley's prophecy of this in *Brave New World*, in which workers were "trained" to tolerate toxic chemicals.

The expansion of the notion of illness also meets a social need. It allows us to sweep under the social rug whole groups of people who are otherwise a nuisance. They may not seek to be categorised as ill. Indeed they may resist or resent it. But, if doctors are prepared to say that particular forms of behaviour, or merely the incidents of growing old, are indeed illnesses, who are we to protest? The twinge of guilt we may feel about neglecting our fellow men, or even locking them away, is salved by the reassuring knowledge that they are ill and are now in the best possible hands in the circumstances. And, provided we keep our hospitals for the mentally ill and long-stay patients out in the backwoods, and their hostels in the decaying urban centres – indeed, anywhere but in our own particular neighbourhood – we can keep up this fiction. In fact, we have in this way created a separate society for the dispossessed and disadvantaged. Forgotten or underprivileged patients are looked after in these institutions by doctors and nurses from overseas, while the menial work is also done by immigrants – "The underprivileged caring for each other in mutual under-standing", as Michael Wilson puts it in his book *Health is for People*. Or is it mutual resentment? You may be intrigued to learn, by the way, that the domestic running costs, just food, laundry, cleaning and so on, of an average mental hospital are about one-third of those of a London teaching hospital. That many are there in the first place is bad enough; that they should be so shabbily dealt with demon-strates the extent of the neglect.

Let me now turn to the second matter. The point I would make about the notion of illness is that it has, with disease, become the central concern of modern medicine. If we were to start all over again to design a model for modern medicine, most of us, I am sure, would opt for a design which concerned itself far, far more with the pursuit and preservation of health, of well-being. What we have instead is the very opposite: a system of medicine which reacts, which responds, which waits to pick up the broken pieces – a form of medicine, in short, concerned with illness, not health. A moment's thought demonstrates the folly of this. But the interests which combine to produce this state of affairs are too well entrenched for any redirection to be accomplished easily. Nonetheless, the significance of the present state of medicine should not be underestimated. It conditions the way we spend huge sums of money each year, roughly 6 per cent of our gross domestic product. It conditions the way we think of ourselves. It goes to the root of our value system, our cultural and social heritage. Meanwhile, debates go on among the medical profession as to how many doctors we should be producing. Concern is expressed at the threat posed to existing doctors' livelihoods by a possible glut of doctors. No one stops to say that these questions cannot be answered until the far more fundamental question is tackled: what should modern medicine be doing? The report of the Royal Commission on the National Health Service contents itself with the rather Delphic utterance that "the planned output of medical graduates is about right". No clue is offered as to how this conclusion is arrived at. No indication is given that the Royal Commission even understood that what was involved in such a calculation was profound social and political considerations.

Equally, in the United States, the *New York Times* reported on 2 September 1980 that the "Government takes steps to Avert Glut of Doctors". The Graduate Medical Education National Advisory Committee after four years of study has predicted that there will be 59,000 more doctors than needed by 1990 and 130,000 too many by the year 2000. The calculations are based, of course, on the assumption that medicine will continue to take its present form and that use of doctors by the population will be on the same basis as at present. Again, there seems to be no realisation that such calculations are worthless without first considering the question of what role medicine should have. Furthermore, the Committee is able to warn of this glut while at the same time noticing that in certain regions of the country, and in certain types of medical care, especially lower-paying family practice and other primary care, severe shortages of doctors exist. This maldistribution of doctors, this coexistence of plenty with need, must make assertions of an oversupply ring hollow to many. The way in which modern medicine has developed is, in large part, responsible for this. How it is to be solved is a problem for the future. If it is to be solved, it may be that the claim that there are too many doctors will need to be reconsidered. It may be more accurate to say that there are too many doctors doing the wrong things.

These are some of the ways in which medicine has taken the wrong path. They are, of course, painted with the broad brush. It is important to realise that I am not denying that every day up and down the country wonderful things are being done. Despite this, could the nation's health be better, or if not better then no worse, at some gain, financial and social, to the citizenry if medicine took a different form? But the present state of medicine will take some changing. It is cultivated by the medical profession. It flatters the self-esteem of the doctor to see himself as the problem-solving scientist spreading health. The present state of medicine has readily been adopted by a lay public, persuaded naively that herein lies the path to health, and with expectations which may be unwarranted but which are, of course, a product of the claims made by medicine. But, although it seems to satisfy the aspirations of the doctor, as well as the expectations of the public, in the event no one is satisfied.

For a start, the cost of financing medicine in the form it now takes is clearly beyond what we are willing to pay in the form of taxation. We complain if we are asked to forgo anything, but we vote for promises of reduced taxation and reduced public spending. Of course, the dissatisfaction doctors feel, as rising national costs are reflected in their income tax, is tinged with a professional reluctance to countenance any cuts in expenditure on medical care. Indeed, as a group they are voluble, for example, in their demand for the so-called freedom to prescribe, whatever the cost. If drugs were prescribed under their general chemical name rather than under a specific company's brand name, the N.H.S. would make a considerable saving, estimated to be at least £25 million a year by R. Barry O'Brien, in his important series of articles in the *Daily Telegraph* of November 1979. Yet doctors resist such an obvious financial control as an unconscionable interference in their rights. No one seems to stop to ask where such rights come from, if not from us.

It should be said that the GP's position is not an easy one. The Royal Commission reports that they are "subjected to massive pressure from the drug companies. A study in 1974–5 showed that a typical GP may be exposed to over 1,300 advertisements for 250 drugs each month. In 1977 the cost of sales promotion in the United Kingdom by drug companies was about £71 million, most of it aimed at GPs. The relative isolation of many GPs from pharmacologist and clinical colleagues adds to their problems in evaluating this mountain of material." As O'Brien points out, this promotion amounts to a staggering £1,458 for each doctor in Britain. Furthermore, the practice is growing of GPs being offered discounts and bonuses by drug companies to promote certain drugs, as *The Times* of 12 April 1980 notes in its report of a speech by John Kerr, the former President of the Pharmaceutical Society of Great Britain. These practices, he warned, were being reflected in the prescribing habits of some GPs. This is a commonplace in the United States. For instance, in 1974 the Senate Labour and Welfare Committee, chaired by Senator Edward Kennedy, reported that in 1974 drug companies spent an average of between $3,000 and $5,000 on each U.S. physician. This money was spent merely on sales promotion through gifts of such items as pocket calculators, pens, freezers, and televisions. Some of these were outright gifts, some were bonuses to reward doctors for prescribing a particular drug. In addition, the Committee reported that 2,000 million free drug samples were sent to doctors. Indeed, it is not unusual for a U.S. drug company to spend 15–20 per cent of its annual sales revenue on promotion and advertising, a proportion considerably larger than non-drug companies. In the United Kingdom also, 15 per cent of sales revenue on average is devoted to promotion while between 7 and 12 per cent is spent on research and development.

Equally, doctors are the first to urge the acquisition of ever more expensive equipment. Also, albeit with less stridency, they can be heard arguing the need for better conditions for hospital patients. And finally, of course, when it comes to their pay, they have not been slow to keep themselves at or near the head of the professional league, while at the same time insisting on the right to private practice in addition. The bitter comment attributed to Aneurin Bevan, the Minister of Health in the post-war Government, that to win over the consultants to the cause of the National Health Service he had "choked their mouths with gold", echoes down the years.

A second reason for dissatisfaction with the state of modern medicine is that we, the public, have been led to expect too much and have been more than willing partners in the process. We have come almost to believe in magic cures and the waving of wands. The reality is a constant disappointment. The promised or expected cures are not there. We are also disappointed for another reason. The simple fact is that for large numbers of people the many and varied services offered by medicine are just not available. And I do not mean here the interventionist, hospital-based medicine I have criticised. I mean the preventive and primary care which large segments of the population do not have ready access to and which, if it were accompanied by other appropriate social measures, would help them pursue and enjoy more healthy lives. I will return to this theme at much greater length later. Now, I will merely refer you to the 1979 Report of the Royal Commission on the Health Service which makes the general point most clearly:

"In some declining urban areas and in parts of London in particular the National Health Service is failing dismally to provide an adequate primary care system to its patients."
"Since the establishment of the N.H.S.," the Report goes

on, "the position of those in social classes 4 and 5 appears to have worsened relative to those in social classes 1 and 2."

Now more than ever, wealthier means healthier. Indeed, it is hard to criticise those who argue that the structure of medical education and health care is organised so as to legitimate a form of society in which concern for the weak may be expressed but is translated into action in a fashion which is limited at best. Illness, then, on this analysis, is not a consequence of poverty, wretched living conditions and unfulfilled lives. Illness is separate from and causes these. As Frederick Gates, the first Director of the Rockefeller Foundation, wrote, "misery is a technical not a social problem". Medicine can thus be conceived of as an apolitical, value-free enterprise, a technical enterprise unrelated to the political circumstances of the society in which it is practised. Inequalities or injustices become problems for others, if problems at all, while medicine goes on its blinkered way.

A final reason for dissatisfaction is the role the doctor finds himself playing. Reality casts him in a far different role from the one which he has been trained to expect and perform. A tension is produced between the model and the reality. It has severe repercussions on the morale of many doctors. Take the general practitioner. A large part of his daily clientele are people who quite simply are unhappy. In the absence of anyone else to go to, and in view of the ready availability of the general practitioner and the extended notion of illness cultivated by doctors, the unhappy person diagnoses himself as ill and then goes to his GP. But many GPs feel they are trained to treat those who are "really ill". This is what those years of white coats and science have prepared them for. They think their time is being wasted and, more significantly, they feel impotent in the face of the unhappiness being complained of.

A 1977 survey, by Cartwright and Anderson, referred to in the Royal Commission's Report, showed that a third of all recently qualified GPs felt that they should not have to deal with their patients' family problems and that it was not appropriate for people to seek such help from their GPs. To do something, the doctor commonly prescribes tranquillisers. With the other regularly used mood-changing drugs, these account for about 10 per cent of all prescriptions. Indeed, even the makers of Valium, Hoffman-La-Roche, hardly famous for public-spiritedness, were constrained last August to advise doctors in the United States not to prescribe it for the ordinary stresses of life (whatever that may mean), and similar Department of Health guidelines were published last March in the *British Medical Journal*. As I have already indicated, the GP finds himself playing the part of socialising agent, ensuring that, whatever form the unhappiness or dissatisfaction take, they are kept in check, and whatever pain there is, it is not felt, even if this means that the social and economic conditions which give rise to them remain unaddressed. Alternatively, the GP finds himself faced by those beset by today's common ills. He is in danger of becoming the victim of his own hyperbole, in that he is asked to work wonders when there are none to work. The damage has been done. There are only symptoms to ease, parts to patch. The frustration is inevitable.

Then consider the doctors who work in hospital. If traumatic injury and perhaps some aspects of obstetrics are put aside, hospitals are now largely engaged in two tasks, neither of which remotely conforms to the image of modern medicine represented by the teaching hospital. One task is that of serving as dumping-grounds for the old and so-called mentally ill. The hospital is little more than a hotel or hostel. The frustration of the doctor, trained to see himself not as a carer but as a solver, is obvious and it can only increase as the elderly come to form an even greater proportion of the population. Indeed, quite whether doctors, as trained at present, have a role to play at all in such hospitals, or whether others could not do the job just as well, is a question which presses for an answer.

The other task doctors in hospitals are performing, is that

of calling upon more and more complex and expensive technology to respond to situations in which, when one looks at the general overall picture, there is usually little that can be done. To use the metaphor of the mechanic, the tyre can be patched, but even so it is permanently weak. I know well that there are some who will say, "It is all very well talking in general terms, but I have got Mr A who is clamouring for help, or Miss B whom I may be able to help. Then there is old Mrs C's hip operation, and Mr D's hernia to fix. I cannot tell them to think of the generality of care, I have a duty to them."

I concede much of this. But let me make two points. First, I am not advocating we burn down our hospitals tomorrow. Of course, we need our marvellous accident units, our general medicine and surgery, whether it be for hips or hernias, haemorrhoids or Hodgkin's disease. But, even here, I wonder how much more rewarding and beneficial it would be to work towards preventing, for example, the degeneration of the hip, or to concentrate on other preventive measures, such as a production system which does not give productivity bonuses, nor uses piece-rates, in industries in which these are known to be associated with an increase in work accidents. How much more rewarding these measures would be than to have units waiting to pick up the pieces and work wonders in sewing the parts together so that the seams are barely visible. If such preventive strategies as these were pursued, greater attention could be paid to the marvellous developments, for example in aiding those with ailing sight or hearing, where the benefits conferred are more than short-term or palliative and where the numbers who could be helped are so great.

My second point is that, put baldly, certain services simply should not be offered until matters of greater priority are dealt with. We have to meet head on the sort of argument advanced in a recent letter to *The Times* from a doctor. "A dying man", Dr Jessop wrote, "does not care that facilities can only benefit a tiny fraction of those patients whose lives might be salvaged. The chance of being among them is all he's got." There are perfectly respectable ethical theories which, in the context of harsh choices, such as those we face now (and always will as regards resources), allow for conduct which will benefit the larger or more worthy number, even if this inevitably means others may suffer. One example, was the decision taken by the U.S. Surgeon-General in the Second World War in North Africa that only those who, on recovery, would be able to fight again should receive scarce penicillin. Thus, those "wounded" in brothels received penicillin; those wounded badly in military engagements did not. Another is the decision now being taken in Uganda to feed only those starving children who may recover, leaving the rest to die.

Our situation is not so desperate, but the same principle must apply. Indeed, such decisions are made every day in the National Health Service when resources come to be allocated. As Michael Wilson, a doctor and theologian, argued recently, in his book *Health is for People*, "only when we are prepared to let some people die will we be free to make more humane decisions in the distribution of resources. Our fear of death leads us to use death as the final incontrovertible argument." We are prepared to ignore much human misery for the prospect of saving a few lives. John James, Assistant Secretary at the Department of Health and Social Security in charge of planning, remarked recently that consultants opposed to shifts of resources from the well endowed areas to the Cinderella areas of geriatrics and mental illness have not been averse to using "shroud-waving tactics".

Well, after these rather harsh words about the wrong emphasis adopted by modern medicine, the wrong path it has taken, I shall consider in the next chapter how the emphasis should be shifted – what a better path for the future may be.

3
Suffer the little children

IT is hard to avoid the grave conclusion that the National
Health Service has failed us. Certainly, it has failed to
take its opportunities. It must be our task to make it clear
to government, and those who manage and control medicine, that we are not content to watch our health-care services merely tick over at their present level, far less to watch
them slowly disintegrate. There can be and must be
improvement and it is our responsibility to ensure that it
happens.

The provision of health care rests on political and social
decisions. The political values which are supposed to be at
the heart of any decisions made for the provision of health
care are well known – that need should be the sole criterion
of receipt of service and that funds should be raised on the
basis of ability to contribute. Though these values have not
been formally rejected as principles, commitment to them
has certainly wavered. Indeed, the provision of health care
in practice has seen a systematic and widespread departure
from them. What I propose to put before you is a blueprint
for change. It represents an attempt to reassert our faith in
these principles, by adopting measures which will go a long
way towards seeing them become reality.

Before I go on, let me point to the forces which stand

against change and improvement. We have already noticed some of the ways in which modern medicine has taken the wrong path. With the decline of serious threats to health from infections, our health-care system has turned away from environmental considerations towards the notion of personal health care. It has become an illness service rather than a health service. This is not to say that modern health care can do nothing for us; it can, and does, provide many much-needed services. But it could do far, far more if a different balance were struck, a balance which would make it more properly a health service.

The present political climate is a further obstacle to improvement. A time of major economic difficulties would seem an inappropriate one in which to recommend improvement in the health services, if only because it is assumed that improvements would cost money. This is, of course, not necessarily so. For instance, money spent in reducing the number of accidents at work or on the road is money gained in terms of reduced hospital and health-care use, in reduced social security payments and increased economic productivity. What is more, this preoccupation with costs suggests that money is the only value. That it is important is clear, that it is the only value is nonsense.

Next, modern medicine has come to recognise that a large measure of modern illness which is not related to genetic disability is the product of our behaviour and our environment. The main causes of chronic illness and death are heart and respiratory ailments, cancer and strokes, with accidents contributing a large share also. Cigarette smoking, alcohol consumption, appalling dietary habits, dangerous work-places and roads are heavily implicated. Unable to do anything about these conditions, government and medical men have resorted to the apologia that they cannot do anything till people change. This has been called the syndrome of "blaming the victim". For example, the last resort of those faced with the carnage of lung cancer is to say, "We have done our best. We have shown the link between smoking and cancer of the lung. It is just that people will not stop smoking." People are castigated as feckless or irresponsible. They eat the wrong foods. They drink too much. Pregnant women will not use the antenatal services available. People just will not take care of themselves. This may appear to let medicine off the hook, but what is lost, or ignored, is the fact that the victim, the one whose life patterns are responsible for his illness, is a product of his environment and often can do little to shape or control it. You can only make the right choices as to food or lifestyle if you have the proper information, if you have the appropriate health education from an early age, and if you have the power or capacity to implement your choice.

These are some of the obstacles in the way of reshaping and improving our health care. They are the product of political and economic decisions and circumstances. So, if there is to be any improvement, it will come only through major political, social and economic changes.

Let me now put before you what I see as the necessary requirements for a reorientation of our health care – a blueprint, if you will. First, the mere provision of more and more money will not of itself improve the quality of our health care. Unfavourable comparisons have been made between the proportion of gross domestic product spent in the United Kingdom on health care, and that spent by the United States or West Germany. In 1977, the proportion was 5.6 per cent in the United Kingdom as against 6.7 per cent in Germany and 7.4 per cent in the United States. By 1979, the U.S. proportion had grown with startling rapidity to over 9 per cent. Both Germany and the United States also had proportionately more doctors that the United Kingdom. But the Royal Commission on the National Health Service cautions against using such comparisons as the basis for any "sweeping assertions". For example, the latest available figures show that both West Germany and the United States, despite their greater expenditure on health care, have a worse record in terms of perinatal and maternal mortality than

England and Wales and no better record in life expectancy.

It is trite to remark that it is not the amount of money but how it is spent which is significant. If, for example, we continue to think of health care in terms which give pride of place, as regards resources, to hospitals, we could easily find ourselves spending more and more, with no great benefit to the overall health of the nation. Furthermore, as members of the Unit for the Study of Health Policy, at Guy's Hospital, London, argue in their 1978 pamphlet, *The NHS in the next 30 years*, short-term increases in financial outlay may well be offset by longer-term financial gain produced by reduced use of health care resources by a healthier population, increased productivity and prosperity, and reduced rates of crime and vandalism.

Second, we must curb our predilection for medicine in the form of ever more complex technology. Note, I do not say abandon it. But we must keep it and its advocates, doctors and commercial entrepreneurs, under our control. Hospitals with their massive costs, expensive equipment and commitment to technology have elbowed themselves into the centre of the medical stage, consuming now some 70 per cent of available health-care resources. The debate in the United Kingdom during the autumn of 1980 concerning the merits of heart transplants offers a useful lesson. It has been carried on largely by doctors, as if what was at stake was a narrow technical matter, instead of a profound question as to the proper direction of our health-care resources. In reality, heart transplants are only an example, and, because of their rarity and relative uselessness, virtually an irrelevance. There are after all 400 deaths a day in the United Kingdom from heart disease. The real debate is much wider. It concerns advanced technology, interventionist, last-ditch, patch-and-repair medicine as against other measures aimed at reducing the need for such intervention. The debate should not be in terms of "either . . . or". It must be in terms of "How much of each do we need and can we afford?"

Quite clearly, we need, and have come to rely on, medical technology in the treatment of kidney disease, in aiding the blind and deaf, in avoiding the birth of deformed and disabled babies and in many other areas. What we do not need, and must guard against, is a mentality which conceives of medical care only, or primarily, in terms of such technological approaches. Instead we need to direct more of our energy and resources towards the promotion of good health. One tragic but often overlooked feature of the defence of heart transplant surgery is that it is so clearly an example of the crazy contradictions of our society. We can only transplant hearts if we have otherwise healthy corpses from which to take them. Where do we get such corpses? We depend on the appalling death rate from road accidents, most of which are eminently preventable.

I now pass to the third point in this blueprint for the future shape of medicine. One of the declared aims of the reorganisation of the National Health Service in 1974 was the integration of individual with community care. The result has been less than successful. Primary care is on the verge of collapse in some areas. Where it functions, it may not be meeting the real needs of the community. If GPs were more adequately prepared for the real health needs of their patients, which are as much to do with social problems as with particular diseases, then the beginnings of a move-ment towards better health could emerge. Progress is undoubtedly being made now that post-graduate training for those intending to be GPs is widespread and will become compulsory by 1981. Indeed, the GP could well become an important focus for the sort of social reform necessary to produce the improvement in health we claim we desire. No one is better placed to gauge the social pressures and problems of the day and pass the news on up the line, and no one is better placed to act as an educator for better health and pass the word down the line.

Besides the primary care of the GP, there is the need for greater emphasis on community medicine. The reorganisa-

tion of the National Health Service introduced on All Fools'
Day 1974, as H.A Waldron notes in his book *The Medical
Role in Environmental Health*, destroyed the long tradition of
the much valued medical officer of health and launched the
newly created community physicians on uncharted seas.
They soon became sucked into administration and are
largely concerned with personal care rather than public
health. The net result has been unfilled posts, disenchant-
ment, and reluctance of newly qualified doctors to go
anywhere near the job. The decline of community medicine
in training and as a career has meant that half the present
community physicians were qualified before 1950 and three-
quarters before 1955. And in a study published in 1976, in
the *British Medical Journal*, by J. Parkhouse and C.
McLaughlin, out of 2,022 newly qualified doctors, only 10
put community medicine as their first choice for a career.
Yet no one can really doubt that a substantial contribution
to health could be made by someone whose job it is, as
community physicians in Oxford put it in their evidence to
the Royal Commission on the N.H.S., to be responsible for
"highlighting the health problems in his particular population, for stimulating different health professionals to plan
their services to meet these problems, and for evaluating and
monitoring the success of these services".

One example may make the point. Claims that hospital
use has been reduced and money thereby saved by the
earlier discharge of patients, particularly the elderly and
mentally ill, ring hollow if on examination it is clear that the
services in the community which are then supposed to take
over are just not adequate to the task, so that the patient
must be re-admitted or languish alone and neglected.

This same understaffing and general demoralisation is
reflected in other areas of community health. The school
health services are woefully ill equipped to engage in the
kind of thorough preventive care and health education
which would pay such dividends in the child's later life. The
Report of the Court Committee on Child Health Services in

1976 drew particular attention to the "failure of the school health service to give adequate attention to health education". Occupational health is another example of a missed opportunity. Its aim is to promote health at work and thereby reduce accidents and injuries. It is a subject which is neglected in medical training. As Waldron points out, there are only 46 specialist industrial doctors per million male workers. Under the Departmental umbrella of the Department of Employment and separated from the National Health Service, occupational health and safety stumble along while accidents at work kill 650 people a year and an estimated million are injured and require time off.

It follows, then, and this is my next point, that, important as the emphasis on primary and community care may be, even greater emphasis must be placed by our health service in the future on two interrelated exercises – the prevention of illness and accidents and the promotion of health. Since I lay great stress on this, let us be clear from the beginning what I am saying. I do not see preventive care as some panacea for all our ills. Furthermore, I readily concede, as I have already said, that we need, and must not neglect, many of our existing medical services. I do not advocate that we become therapeutic nihilists, and decry everything that goes by the name of medicine today. Indeed, as Muir Gray points out in his book *Man Against Disease*, some take the view that prevention has three phases. First, you can prevent disease – primary prevention. Then you can prevent the effects of disease, by treatment at an early stage – secondary prevention. And, third, you can prevent the serious consequences of disease by further treatment – tertiary prevention. Curative medicine may be concerned with prevention at the secondary and tertiary stages. So it is not a question of *either* curative medicine *or* preventive medicine, as some would make it seem. It is rather a question of where along the spectrum you concentrate most resources.

In my view, for us to have a sane health care policy, we

must concentrate much more on primary preventive medicine. If this means, as it inevitably must, that some aspects of modern curative care must be neglected or abandoned, then so be it. The benefits to be gained outweigh any loss. It will mean that profound changes will have to be made. The mentality adopted towards medical care, illness and health by doctors and laymen alike must change, research must redirect itself, at least in part, and resources must be reallocated on a considerable scale. That the chapter in the Royal Commission's Report on the National Health Service which dealt with these issues was the shortest, bar one, in the whole Report suggests that the process of change may not be easy.

A first essential step in any process towards redirecting effort or reallocating resources is to see how these are at present distributed. It is no rhetorical device to describe the disparities in the present provision of health care among the various groups in our society as a scandal. The evidence has been available for a long time. *Inequalities in Health*, the 1980 report compiled by a group under the chairmanship of Sir Douglas Black, President of the Royal College of Physicians, is the latest and most impressive account to appear. In the dry language of such reports, the group found "marked inequalities in health between the social classes in Britain". At birth and in the first month of life, the death rate of babies born to parents in social class 5, the unskilled, is double that of babies born to parents in social class 1, professional workers. In the next eleven months, four times as many boys and five times as many girls in class 5 die, as in class 1. Compared with class 1, men in class 5 have twice the rate of long-standing illness, women in class 5 two and a half times the rate. A baby born of class 1 parents can expect to live 5 years longer on average than a child of class 5 parents. If class 4 (the semi-skilled) and class 5 had had the same mortality rates as class 1 in 1970–2 (the latest years for which there are reliable figures), 74,000 people, including 10,000 children, would not have died. Indeed, if a line were drawn from the Wash to the Bristol Channel those living north of the line, the large majority of whom are members of classes 4 and 5, have on average a shorter lifespan and higher disease rates than those south of the line.

J. Tudor Hart writes of an "inverse care law" which provides that where there is most sickness and death GPs have the largest number of patients, the heaviest work load and the least hospital support. The 1979 Report of the Royal Commission on the National Health Service noted bleakly that in terms of health "the position of those in social classes 4 and 5 appears to have worsened relative to those in social classes 1 and 2 since the inception of the National Health Service in 1948", though it goes on to point out that all social classes are healthier than thirty years ago. This makes the almost contemptuous dismissal of Sir Douglas Black's report by the present Secretary of State hard to understand. The Secretary of State admits "disappointment" that there is generally little sign of health inequalities diminishing. But, he goes on, additional expenditure, on the scale which could result from the recommendations of this report could be upwards of £2 billion a year. This, he concludes, is quite unrealistic. The cost point is not argued, nor, it seems, is any account taken of possible short- or long-term savings and benefits which would accrue to a country whose people are healthier. And no account at all is taken of values other than monetary ones, the most obvious being the sheer injustice of operating a system which fails to meet its stated aim, the provision of health care with equality of entitlement and access.

So change and improvement are hardly around the corner. But this does not deter me from offering my views. And, if political action is called for, political education is a first and necessary stage. So let us consider some specific aspects of this part of the blueprint, the need to emphasise the prevention of accidents and illness and the promotion of health.

One argument put forward by those anxious to maintain the existing emphasis on interventionist medicine is that you cannot prevent illness, or promote health, until you know what causes illness or ill health. And, to discover causes, you need the sort of medicine practised now, backed by technology and research. There is, of course, some truth in this. The argument goes on that we simply do not yet know what causes the common illnesses which afflict and kill us, with perhaps the exceptions of smoking and its relationship with lung cancer, and alcohol with liver damage. The implication is that, until we do, medicine should continue in its present form. Consider the fact that in the United States mortality from heart disease has declined in recent years, concurrently with an increase in exercise and a great reduction in smoking. Yet arguments about the role played by eating fat, or exercising, or smoking, in heart disease still continue. Indeed, if we are to wait until the perfect controlled experiment has demonstrated that it is factor X which is the real killer, preventive medicine will have to await the millennium. Besides, it must be obvious by now that research aimed at isolating individual causative agents is of doubtful validity, since there are few modern afflictions which can be traced to one particular cause. There are after all good historical precedents for taking action to prevent illness without the ability to justify the action scientifically. When in 1853 John Snow removed the handle of the Broad Street water pump in Soho, he could not prove the link between the water and cholera. Indeed, the prevailing theory was that cholera was carried by foul air. But, once the pump handle was removed, the cholera did not spread. Equally, we can now observe that people who are obese seem more prone to illness, and most of us know what makes us fat. Indeed, insurance underwriters, those most hard-headed of people, follow a simple rule. The more overweight you are, the higher the premium they demand. They do not await definitive, scientific proof. So, while I concede the value of some modern interventionist medicine, in terms of the information and insights it may offer, this does not persuade me that it must be supported in all its various forms, or that preventive care must necessarily play second fiddle to it.

My second specific point is one which must already be clear. To reorient health care towards prevention and health promotion, political will and political action are crucial requirements. As Sir George Young, the Under-Secretary of State at the Department of Health, said recently at a Conference in Stockholm, "For many of today's medical problems, the answer may not be cure by incision at the operating table, but prevention by decision at the Cabinet table." Aaron Wildavsky makes the same point when he states that "According to the Great Equation, medical care equals health. But the Great Equation is wrong . . . The best estimates are that the medical system affects about 10 per cent of the usual indices for measuring health . . . the remaining 90 per cent are determined by factors over which doctors have little or no control, from individual life style . . to social conditions . . . to the physical environment."

This brings me to my next point. To establish the basis for the promotion and pursuit of health as well as the prevention of illness, there must be a commitment to education. We need, quite simply, to learn how to live healthy lives or, even more fundamentally, we need to have the opportunity to learn. Such education has two roles. It must combat what Professor J. N. Morris, in his paper in the *British Medical Journal*, of 19 January 1980, called "the multi-million pound anti-health forces" – the tobacco, alcohol and food industries, and their advertisers, who bombard us with misinformation. And there is positive education, which must begin in schools and be carried on in office, workplace and in the home. The government-established Health Education Council commands the pathetically puny sum of £4½ million a year in pursuit of a task which is central to health care. For example, it must try to educate us of the dangers of cigarette smoking on about £½ million a year while the tobacco industry spends £70 million extolling the pleasures of smoking. Health visitors, nurses who spend a further year of study in preventive medicine, also have a central role to play, which they discharge with great dedication. But there are too few of them, and, as the Royal Commission on the N.H.S. pointed out, training oportunities are inadequate. Equally, the Commission highlighted the need for more health education officers, whose job it is to promote adult health education. In 1977 there were a mere 300 for the whole of Britain. Doctors too have a role to play in this educative process, whether in the surgery or out-patient department, whether about diet or accidents in the home.

But, according to Professor McKeown, it is a major problem to get doctors to think in terms of the community, the environment, preventive care and the promotion of health, as against the diagnosis and treatment of established disease.

Public education can, of course, come through the medium of the press, radio and television. Consider how much attention is given by these to strikes, and even threats of strikes, as imperilling our national well-being through lost working days. I am certainly not saying this should not be reported and I concede that strikes can have drastic effects. Over the last decade an average of 13 million working days have been lost each year through strikes. But where is the headline and leader column and news flash and interview concerning tooth decay, which accounts for an average of 4 million lost working days a year, costs the N.H.S. £200 million a year, and is entirely preventable? Where is the special report on television or in the press on the causes of back pain, which accounts for about 18 million lost working days a years, at a cost to the N.H.S. of £900 million, and could be greatly reduced through proper education? And where is the outcry in the press against injuries at work, which account for an estimated 48 million lost working days a year? Is it too much to hope that the press will at last discover that one-tenth of all lost working days are the result of bronchitis, which kills 30,000 people a year, costs several hundreds of millions of pounds in N.H.S. costs, as well as lost productivity and social security payments, yet could be greatly reduced if cigarette smoking were curbed? Is it too much to hope that there will be some rethinking in Fleet Street as to what is really "the English disease"?

My third specific point is that any concern for preventive care or the promotion of health must include a strategy for confronting the threat posed by the major destroyers of our day. These are, of course, cigarettes, alcohol, poor diet and accident (whether at home, on the roads, or at work), and here I am not talking about education concerning these threats but rather about the need to take some action. We simply have to do better than we have done, so far, in controlling these scourges.

Take cigarette smoking first. The Government of the day had its first meeting with the tobacco industry some twenty-three years ago. Yet cigarette advertisements are still all about us. Meanwhile 1,000 die prematurely each week from the effects of cigarette smoking. About 1,500 babies die each year, and many more are handicapped, because their mothers smoked during pregnancy. Despite the hundreds of millions of pounds spent here and elsewhere on the pursuit of treatment and cure for lung cancer, in the true traditions of modern scientific medicine, and with little or no success, relatively little work has been carried out by medical researchers (as opposed to advertisers) to discover why people smoke, and how they can be helped to stop. Only in May 1980 the Secretary of State at the D.H.S.S. announced in Parliament that his Ministry was to sponsor research into the motives and pressures causing people, especially the young, to smoke. He expected, he said, that the report would be available by the end of 1981. Why, it could be asked, has it taken so long to commission such research, particularly in view of the increase in cigarette smoking documented by Lesley Doyal in her outstanding book, *The Political Economy of Health*? Between 1958 and 1975 there was an increase in smoking of 9 per cent for men and a startling 63 per cent for women in class 5, with a consequent increase in death from lung cancer, while in class 1 there was a fall of 53 per cent for men and 15 per cent for women.

One cause of reluctance to take on the tobacco industry stems, of course, from the tangled economic arguments. It is estimated that between 4 and 5 per cent of government revenue comes from tobacco sales tax. In 1975 the *New Scientist* reported that a "grisly analysis" had been carried out by the Health Department, showing that "a reduction in smoking would eventually cost the country more than was gained; not only would there be loss of revenue from taxation but also the additional 'burden' of having to pay out pensions to the people who had given up smoking before it killed them". And of course there are about 30,000 jobs in the tobacco industry to consider, not to mention the £11½ million that newspapers derive from advertisements and the livelihood of corner shopkeepers.

These are the arguments which support the *status quo*. I would make two comments. First, any economic analysis is so extraordinarily hard to carry out that such conclusions as those arrived at by the Health Department must be viewed with great suspicion. Second, there are, of course, values other than money, such as happiness and health, which should not be ignored and which, even in the case of a purely economic analysis, would significantly affect the conclusions arrived at. I hardly need stress that the economic indicator of productivity is much affected by the health and sense of personal satisfaction of the workforce.

Then there is our diet. The food industry, as Doyal again ably demonstrates, has been enormously successful in ruining our diet, and consequently our health. For example, more and more food is made from raw materials which have been refined. Look at bread. The ordinary loaf of white bread is not lacking in nutrition. What it lacks is bulk. This lack encourages overconsumption. Overconsumption sells more bread and so produces greater profits. It also produces obesity and the consequent threat to health. And the story has a twist in the tail. The food industry has gone on to develop a second string to its bow, the sale of health foods and vitamin tablets. To make up for what has been removed from some food by its being processed and refined, vitamins and health foods – which are, of course, more expensive than ordinary food – then appear on the market. Thus, the wealthier can get the food they need, since they can afford to buy it. The poor cannot and another inroad into health promotion and the prevention of illness is made. Another example Doyal refers to is the successful campaign to persuade mothers to use modified cow's milk rather than breast-feed their babies. Not only does the baby fail to obtain immunities gained through mother's milk, but mothers are also encouraged to switch from bottle-feeding to commercially prepared solid food as soon as possible, despite the fact that this contributes to child obesity. So successful was the campaign that by the mid-1970s only about 6 per cent of mothers in the United Kingdom breast-fed their babies.

As regards accidents, in addition to the 650 killed at work each year, there are a further 6,500 deaths from accidents in the home and at play. Each week 100 miners suffer disabling injuries, yet the occupational health service continues to be neglected. Despite the annual carnage on the roads of about 75,000 people injured and 7,500 killed, only a third of drivers wear safety belts. Furthermore, in the case of children in cars it is estimated that 85 per cent of the deaths and 70 per cent of the injuries would have been prevented if the child had been restrained. Yet opposition to the compulsory wearing of seat belts still appears to be winning the day.

The Parliamentary Secretary at the Ministry of Transport told Parliament on 18 December 1980 that the Health Service would save between £6 million and £7 million a year if seat belts were worn by all front seat occupants. The taxpayer would be saved a further £10 million a year in social security benefits. And lost productive output which would be saved had, he said, been estimated at £100 million a year. But despite such huge potential savings, around £117 million a

year, he refused to be drawn on whether the government
had plans to make the wearing of seat belts compulsory.

The story of alcohol is similar to that of cigarettes. The
Health Education Council spends about £½ million publi-
cising the health dangers of alcohol, while about £36 million
is spent advertising its pleasures by the industry. According
to a Report of the Royal College of Physicians, published in
March 1980, we are already experiencing an epidemic of
alcoholism. Besides causing cirrhosis, the number of deaths
from which has doubled to 2,000 a year in the past twenty
years, alcohol is also implicated in such illnesses as cancer,
heart disease and strokes. Equally, it is linked to the
incidence of crime, domestic violence and absenteeism.
And, of course, its effect on driving is well known. An estimated 30 per cent of road accident deaths are the result of
someone driving while incapable through alcohol. Among
young people, it is estimated to be the principal cause of
road accident deaths. The immediate preventive effect of the
Road Traffic Act 1967 was enormous, saving an estimated
1,000 lives in the first year after it became law. But things
have become progressively worse. Despite spending by
government of large sums of money, £500,000 in 1977
alone, seeking to persuade drivers not to drink and drive,
the problem seems only to be worse. The case is surely
made for stronger government action.

Of course, it is fair to note that there are those who, when
faced with the prospect of seat belt legislation, or increased
taxes on cigarettes or alcohol, will argue that there is a limit
to the extent to which government should (not can, but
should) interfere in the life of the individual. When
Chadwick, the pioneer of public health legislation, had his
legislation defeated in 1854 and disappeared from public life,
The Times thundered, "We prefer to take our chance with
cholera, than to be bullied into health." There is much that
is cant and unreason in such calls for individual freedom,
even though there is also a perfectly respectable philosophical argument. For, in today's society, there is little an

individual can do which does not impinge on others. The smoker, for example, draws sickness pay, receives medical care and dies in hospital, all funded from public revenue. When he cannot work, he and his dependents are supported from public funds. Equally, the driver or passenger who fails to wear his seat belt is treated in the intensive care unit and recuperates in hospital at a high cost to the public purse. And if he dies or cannot work he and his family live off public funds.

Let us consider next two other threats to health, often overlooked. They are unemployment and the level of subsistence available to those who must rely on social security benefits. Unemployment has of course a number of devastating effects, not least the loss of a sense of worth and the consequent desperation or frustration. Unemployment also threatens health in the sense that family income and consequent levels of nutrition and quality of housing and recreation are affected adversely. Harvey Brenner, in a now famous study at Johns Hopkins University in the United States, has shown that the increase in U.S. unemployment between 1970 and 1975 of 1¼ million people was responsible for an extra 26,000 deaths from heart and kidney disease, 5,500 extra admissions to mental hospitals, 1,700 extra homicides, 1,500 extra suicides and 900 extra deaths from cirrhosis, through excessive consumption of alcohol. Studies in Australia and here in the United Kingdom bear out this thesis. Furthermore, as a task force of the U.S. Department of Health, Education, and Welfare reported in 1973, "in an impressive 15 year study of aging, the strongest predictor of longevity was work satisfaction". Such arguments lend a cutting edge to polite political debate about the regrettable level of unemployment.

Equally, those who live on social security benefits constantly teeter on the brink of ill health. Already, many of the elderly and disabled live in a state of relative poverty. Already, many of them have difficulty in meeting the costs of keeping warm in winter, living as they do in substandard

housing. And with cold comes ill health and, to some,
death. Limit further the resources available to them and the
risks only grow. Already, many are socially isolated and
subsist on the barest minimum of food. With malnutrition
comes ill health and, to some, death. Limit further the
resources available and the risks only grow.

This leads me to my fourth point in this consideration of
preventive care and the promotion of health. Such action as
there is on the part of government seems bedevilled by a
confusion of aims and complexity of organisation. Nowhere
is this more true than in the case of the provision made for
environmental health.

As H. A. Waldron points out, "The main problem
relating to environmental health is . . . the fragmentation of
services . . . there is expertise in abundance . . . but it is
scattered haphazardly throughout many different organisations and institutions." As the issues become more
complex, the mechanisms for response, through their
complexity, become less able to meet the need. "Consider
the control of pesticides," Waldron suggests. "In England,
no less than nine departments are involved to some degree,
in Scotland, three, whilst the Welsh Office protects some of
the Welsh interests. . . . With so many thumbs in the pie",
he concludes, "it is not difficult to see that the right boy
may not always get the plum."

What is also remarkable in the approach of government to
the issue of health promotion is the apparent inability, or
unwillingness, to see how interrelated are so many of the
various decisions of government departments, both national
and local. When considering the allocation of resources, it is
assumed that claims for spending on, for example, housing
or industry or transport or social security compete with
claims for spending on health. In fact, of course, they may
all be involved in the same exercise. Savings on social
services often mean inevitable increases in health expenditure. Take the decision of the Minister of Transport, in
1977, to restore the maximum speed limit to 70 miles per

hour, despite the demonstrable reduction, by 14 per cent, in the number of people killed or injured on the roads between 1973 and 1975, when the speed limit was lower. Some of the reduction may have been due to the fact that cars were used less because of the increased petrol prices, but even allowing for this the Minister's decision had as an effect the promotion of accidents rather than of health, and consequently increased the costs borne by the N.H.S.. Equally, any rise or fall in the cost, in real terms, of the tax levied on the sale of alcohol will directly affect the numbers of people maimed and killed by drunken drivers.

Local authority spending cut-backs, prompted by loss of national government grants, may well lead to increased spending by national government, if the elderly or disabled have to be admitted to hospital, because the money for such services as home helps, warm meals, social workers, or sheltered housing is no longer there. Decisions in the Industry or the Employment Departments, whether they concern the number of safety inspectors in factories or the level of unemployment, affect directly the promotion or otherwise of health, and consequently the extent of the call on the National Health Service's resources.

Considerations such as these seem to get lost in the scramble by government departments for budgets, and the desire for profit or loss in one department's book, whatever the overall picture. Each department has its separate brief, its separate policy goals, and, most important, its separate budget. Some properly institutionalised system of co-ordination of policy aimed at promoting health, a goal you would have thought would be a high priority, seems almost entirely lacking. For example, imaginative proposals to employ financial or tax incentives in efforts to improve or promote health, are few and far between. The elderly could be helped to avoid the poverty trap, and its ensuing threat to health, by simple measures such as removing the liability to forfeit social security benefits once earnings rise above a certain sum. The loss of revenue involved would be far outweighed by savings in health and social services spending because of a healthier and happier and more productive elderly population.

Admittedly, the Exchequer has used taxation to some extent as a device to control cigarette consumption, but with considerable ambivalence, given the revenue it derives from the tax on cigarette sales. Remarkably, the cost in real terms of alcoholic beverages has declined in the past decade, despite warnings of an epidemic of alcoholism. Compare the approach by government in France to one problem, that of infant and maternal mortality rates. These have been dramatically reduced, from 22 per cent above the United Kingdom in 1960, to 10 per cent below in 1970, not only because resources were invested in manpower and buildings, but also through the use of such devices as financial benefits made available to pregnant women conditional upon regular attendance at antenatal clinics. Since the infant mortality rate is a good indicator of child health, it is likely that the proportion of handicapped children in the population is now less in France than in the United Kingdom, with consequent savings to the public purse, let alone the increased happiness among the citizenry.

Of all the various proposals for the promotion of health and the prevention of illness, I have left the most important until last. I refer to the health of our children. If we are to improve the health of the nation, we have no choice but to redirect an enormous amount of our resources to the care of children, before birth, at birth, and during their development. If ever there was a case for the promotion of health, this must be it. It is in fact one of the declared priorities of the N.H.S., but little yet has been achieved. Indeed the results are disgraceful. Once again, it has to be realised that what is needed is not just tinkering with or retooling the N.H.S. The result would be cosmetic at best. What is called for is the realisation that the state of our children's health, and thus their and our future, is a consequence of the whole style of our society and that if anything is to be done then some fairly profound political action is called for.

It is a measured understatement to say that as a society we could do more for the health of our children. The problem of course is not new. As J. A. Muir Gray points out, the improvement in the general health of adults at the end of the nineteenth century was not accompanied by improvements in child health. So low was the level of fitness of the British working class that half the young men who volunteered for the Boer War were turned away as unfit. The minimum height for entry into the infantry had to be dropped from 5 feet 6 inches in 1882 to 5 feet in 1902. The shock was such as to provoke the passing of legislation in 1906 and 1907 to establish a school medical and school meal service. The thinking was not, or course, wholly philanthropic or egalitarian. There was also a need for a fitter, more productive labour force.

Our perinatal mortality and morbidity rates in the United Kingdom, the death and sickness rates, compare unfavourably with most other countries of similar economic and social development. And who are the children who are suffering? Let me remind you of the words of Sir Douglas Black's Report, *Inequalities in Health*:

"From the end of the first month to the end of the first year . . . for the death of every 1 male infant in class 1, we can expect . . . 4 deaths in class 5. Among female infants these ratios are even more disadvantageous to the offspring of manual workers."

Perinatal mortality, death of a baby at birth or in the first week of life, accounts for seven babies per thousand in class 1, but 27 in every thousand born into class 5. Antenatal and perinatal care simply are not being delivered to those most in need, those in social classes 4 and 5. Women in these groups, according to Muir Gray, "go to clinic for the first time later in the course of pregnancy, attend less regularly, and follow the advice given less punctiliously. For instance, they more frequently continue to smoke." The reasons are many and include, for example, transport difficulties, the siting of clinics, the need to care for other children, an acquired antipathy to authority, and the middle-class attitudes of doctors, with their emphasis on rationality and planning, not shared by the working class. *The Times* of 15 April 1980 carried the report of the Central Birmingham Community Health Council which highlighted the fact that women most at risk in pregnancy came from the poorest homes and had the least adequate facilities available to them. Indeed, the report showed that in inner-city areas such as Sparkbrook the perinatal mortality rate was 80 per cent higher than the national average. A second study by the West Midlands Regional Health Authority, reported in *The Times* on 6 May 1980, showed that only 21 per cent of pregnant women over forty years of age in this area had recourse to antenatal care, despite their high-risk category.

It is the children of these same families who are no longer immunised against the common infections. Large numbers of parents have, for example, been frightened off by the well-meaning but ill-advised campaign against whooping-cough vaccination. The allegation was that vaccination carried a risk of inducing brain damage in the child. The cause of children who, it was said, had suffered such damage was championed by certain Members of Parliament and the children ultimately received compensation from the State. The proof was not strong, the numbers were very few as compared with the millions who benefited without ill effect, but the cause was popular. The unhappy consequence has been that the attention the campaign attracted caused many mothers to lose confidence in all forms of immunisation for their children, not just against whooping cough. Since then, the United Kingdom has seen a mild epidemic of whooping cough with some few deaths recorded. It may well be that we shall have to undergo the horrors of a polio epidemic before parents will be persuaded once again to avail themselves of this most basic and easily available of preventive measures.

It is these same children in social classes 4 and 5 who do

not receive adequate testing for hearing and sight and whose prospects for educational and emotional development, never the brightest, are handicapped still further. Indeed, the poor services available for the deaf mean that more than half of the children born deaf are not diagnosed until they are at least three years old. Nonetheless, *The Times* of 6 May 1980, reports that, according to the National Deaf Children's Society, teaching services for the deaf are to be cut further by more than a fifth.

It is these same children whose nutrition and health are' most affected by political decisions, made in the name of economy, to raise the price of school meals or abandon the service, to curtail the supply of free school milk, to reduce a whole range of social security benefits, whether supplementary benefits or child benefits or even allowances for childrens' clothing and shoes, to limit access to free school transport, or even dispense with the services and safety afforded by those guardians of the road crossings near schools, the "lollipop ladies". Recall, if you will, that about 5,000 children are killed or injured each year while crossing the road, such that Britain has the worst child pedestrian injury rate in Western Europe.

It is these same children who must live in substandard housing. It is these same children who provide the squalid statistic which has it that 97 per cent of them by the age of 15 will have rotting teeth. Fluoridation of drinking water, which, it has been estimated, would reduce the incidence of dental caries by a half, continues to attract opposition. The Royal Commission on the N.H.S. was moved to conclude that "it is entirely wrong to deprive the most vulnerable section of the population of such an important public health measure, for the sake of the views of a small minority of adults for whom its benefits come too late". But, quite apart from this, the system of dental care negotiated in 1948 at the outset of the N.H.S. makes little or no provision for preventive dentistry. Nor does the elaborate piece-work system of payment encourage it. As Professor Miller puts it, in his book *Medicine and Society*, "the financial basis of professional remuneration might have been specifically designed to produce a cheap and nasty service".

It is these same children who feel the cold wind of unemployment blowing through their parents' lives. It is these same children who will suffer from a mortality rate from accidents five times higher than that of children born into class 1. In sum, the National Child Development Study, which has followed the development of 10,000 children born in the first week of March 1958, demonstrates, in the words of Muir Gray, that the "socially handicapped were shorter in height, more often absent from school, more frequently had hearing loss, more often had a squint, and were twice as likely to have had tuberculosis, meningitis or rheumatic fever. Their housing conditions made . . . the spread of infections more probable." Finally, he notes, "Not surprisingly, the educational achievement of deprived children was lower. One in fourteen of the disadvantaged children was receiving, or waiting to receive, special education compared with one in eighty of those not socially handicapped and educational subnormality was seven times more common."

These inequalities, or iniquities, cannot be shrugged off, yet successive governments seem oblivious. The extent of the re-examination and reorientation of values called for is breathtaking. But so also is the extent of the human wastage and misery, which we tolerate now with hardly a thought as to whether things might be otherwise. By contrast to the magnitude of this task, the squabbling over private medicine, which seems to mesmerise politicians and doctors, is a tragic irrelevance. The Black Report concluded "that the abolition of child poverty should be adopted as a national goal for the 1980s". You will recall the present Secretary of State's thoroughly anaemic comment that the findings of the Black Report on Inequalities in Health will "come as a disappointment to many". They are a disgrace; an indictment of what we are and what we have achieved.

More than 100 years ago Disraeli spoke of our being two nations. We still have not escaped this indictment. Now let those who want to argue about heart transplants do so. It is against this background that the debate must be judged.

In these brief comments, I have sought to sketch the outline of a programme to improve our health care. You may rest assured that those who would oppose it will find reasons of cost to justify doing so. I have little patience with such people. They hide their political choices behind slide rules and balance sheets. My political choices have been made clear. But they are not mine alone. They are what this country purports to stand for. If you begin with them, the figures can come out quite differently. What I have offered is a conceptual framework, not a plan of action. Of course, it calls for action. If we are to change the way in which medicine is thought of and practised, it is we who must take that action. It is our responsibility.

4

"Decisions, decisions . . ."

IN practising medicine doctors routinely make decisions, they make judgements. This much is commonplace. But what sort of judgements or decisions are they? All professionals make judgements. That is what we expect of them. That is what we consult them for. "Leave it to doctor" is an expression which is part of our language, as are such phrases as "doctor's orders" or "doctor knows best". They have, perhaps, been incorporated into our vocabulary without much thought. What are the implications of such language? When we think of doctors' decisions, we think of diagnosis, prognosis, treatment. We think of these decisions as being bounded by and derived from demonstrable objective principles, something called medical expertise. We think of these decisions as matters of technical skill; that is, based on the observation of objective facts and the application of particular skills in the light of such facts. That is what the doctor goes to medical school for, and then spends years on the job learning about. We call these decisions medical decisions. This is what doctors have a special, indeed unique, competence in. But are these matters of technical skill? Do these demonstrable objective principles exist? What are they? What is a medical decision? What is this medical expertise? These may appear to be simple enough questions. But the answers are not so simple, even though they go to the heart of the practice of medicine. Define the nature of a medical decision and you define the role played by doctors.

We could define a medical decision by saying it is one taken by doctors. This cannot be right. The decision as to what vote to cast in a general election is made by doctors, but that does not make it a medical decision. So can we narrow the inquiry down a bit? Can we say it is a decision made by a doctor in a medical context? No, this will not do either. It is circular: what is medical is what is medical. Let us try another approach. Let us say that, in the most general sense, the doctor claims unique competence in making decisions about health and ill health, illness and disease. That is the doctor's *raison d'être*, and it is one accepted by the rest of us. This may satisfy some, but it does not satisfy me. For we have already come to understand that health and illness are not matters of objective reality, on which we all agree, as are, for example, the questions whether humans, generally, have two arms and two legs and one head. Instead, health is a socially determined and evaluative term, just as is its counterpart, ill health. Equally, we have seen that illness is a status – something conferred on someone in the light of particular facts, but not inherent in those facts. The issue is not whether X, objectively, is ill, but whether he ought to be regarded as ill, whether he satisfies certain conditions, which, admittedly, usually include physical realities such as fever or pain (though in the case of mental illness even this requirement is dispensed with), but which also include social, moral and political components, which fall to be considered.

Some of you may protest that this is a caricature, a travesty of the truth. Yes, you may say, doctors certainly make decisions all the time and these do involve judgements, for example how to manage a particular patient. "Manage" is obviously a term involving choices, but, you say, these choices are made by reference to sound medical principles, and out of concern for the patient's best interests. But this still fudges the issue. You still have to tell me what sound medical principles are, and by whom they were developed. You see, my point is that the scope of the alleged unique competence of the doctor is as wide, as imprecise, as flexible and as inherently evaluative as the meanings given to the notions of health and ill health. Doctors make decisions as to what ought to be done. Some, but only some, of these decisions are matters of technical skill. I submit that the majority of decisions taken by doctors are not technical. They are, instead, moral and ethical. They are decisions about what ought to be done, in the light of certain values. Now, this creates a problem. Doctors claim a special, indeed unique, competence in a particular area, the practice of medicine. So medical judgements, medical decisions, are for them and them alone. But, if I am right that it is a fundamental feature of medical practice that doctors are making ethical judgements, it means that ethics, to the extent that they touch on how doctors choose to practise medicine, are something for them, and them alone. This is a surprising and even dangerous notion.

It would normally be accepted that ethical principles, the principles by reference to which we organise our lives and decide what we ought or ought not to do, are not the preserve of any one group. But the doctor may reply that, yes, he does make ethical decisions, but these are medical ethics, and so they are properly for doctors alone. This would suggest that there is a realm of ethics unique to medicine and within the unique competence of doctors to determine and apply. My response is that medical ethics are not separate from, but part of, the general moral and ethical order by which we live. Let me make my point crystal clear. Of course, in one sense, the decisions to be made are for doctors alone to make. They are on the spot, "in the trenches", as it were. I am not suggesting that others should make them. But the decisions must conform to standards set by others. They must be based on principles. Decisions as to what the doctor ought to do must, in short, be tested against the ethical principles of the society. He has no special dispensation to depart from our moral and ethical order. The only special feature of his particular code of ethics can be the obligation to adhere even more strictly than the average citizen to our ethical order, because of the position of power he occupies.

Too often, the moment this debate is opened the floodgates of vitriol are opened also. But the debate should be opened. It must be wrong that power and responsibility in many areas of human concern should be pushed on to doctors by the simple tactic of calling them medical matters, just because we are happy to have others bear this responsibility. Equally, it must be wrong that a doctor, simply by describing a decision as medical, can claim unique competence, and the power which goes with it, to make such a decision, even if it touches the basic values by which we live our lives. For if doctors claim unique competence it must be in something they are uniquely competent to do. Doctors are not uniquely competent to make ethical decisions. They receive no training to prepare them for such a role. So, put rather bluntly, what I am calling for is a wholesale re-examination of the sphere of alleged competence of the doctor.

If you agree with me, as I take you through some examples, that doctors are indeed making ethical decisions in a rather haphazard, idiosyncratic way, then you will want to consider how best we should respond. We may seek to insist, by whatever means is deemed appropriate, that doctors conform to standards and principles set down by all of us. We may suggest that the education of doctors should prepare them more appropriately for the decisions they are called on to make. We may be content merely to remind them that they must look over their shoulders from time to time, to make sure we approve of what they are doing. Some doctors, I am sure, will recognise the truth in what I am suggesting. It is just that they seem to operate on some form of automatic pilot when it comes to matters of ethics. We must gain their attention and provide the correct navigation. There are others, however, who will take more persuading. After all, doctors did not win their dominance in the field of medicine and healing without a struggle; and, having won it, and the power which goes with it, only with the greatest reluctance will an inch of ground be conceded.

Not much more than 100 years ago, those whom we now call doctors competed with many others in the market place of the healing arts. Gradually, scientific medicine won the day in Europe and America. Doctors who chose this new route were licensed and organised themselves into a profession. From such a position of consolidated power, other methods of treating people, other approaches to caring and healing can be denigrated and ostracised as quackery, not only ill conceived, but wrong and possibly harmful. The term "fringe medicine" is used as if there were a central core of proper medical care. Indeed, one of the most interesting social and political conflicts of the next decade will be the challenge to this view.

Take the following propositions. You would not, for example, consider the law of homicide, and exceptions to it, to be a matter for doctors alone to decide upon. Nor would you regard it proper for doctors alone to decide when principles of honesty should be observed or waived. Nor would you regard it properly for doctors alone to decide the appropriate conditions of family life. These are all examples of social and political decisions which go to the root of our culture. Would it surprise you, then, to learn that each is an example of a decision commonly taken by doctors, and regarded as uniquely within their competence to make? And, if it is uniquely within their competence, it follows that only doctors, and no one else, may properly challenge such a decision.

It is doctors who decide whether or not to treat a baby born severely handicapped. It will not die if it receives the

care which babies are ordinarily given. But it will not
prosper. It will always be severely handicapped. It may be
suffering from Down's syndrome – what used to be called
mongolism – or from spina bifida, a condition which, in its
severest form, is attended by gross paralysis of the limbs,
incontinence, the accumulation of fluid in the brain and the
possibility (which cannot be accurately predicted) of the
severest mental handicap.

Let us consider the fate of this spina bifida baby. The
question posed is what to do. The fluid on the brain can be
controlled, and, with a lengthy succession of careful surgical
operations, some of the worst deformities may be corrected,
although function lost cannot be restored. Should this treatment be embarked upon? Perhaps it is as well to know that
if it is not the baby will more than probably die, usually by
recourse to what can best be described as benign neglect.
The baby may be fed only on demand, while given
sedatives which suppress demand. Or the baby may be
nursed, but allowed to succumb to the first infection
without recourse to appropriate medications. An awesome
decision therefore falls to be made. And who makes it? It is
the doctor who makes it. Very often, the parents will be
involved, but I put it to you that this involvement should
not be regarded as significant in terms of the nature of the
decision arrived at, though it may be important in the
process of decision making. This is because parents tend to
do what doctors advise. Even if the doctor purports not to
advise, but merely to state the facts neutrally, nothing is
changed, for it is clear that the choice as to which facts to
present and how to present them will produce the same
result as that produced by more direct advice.

On what criteria does the doctor decide? There are
probably many. Some may reflect his views as to the proper
allocation of resources within the finite amount available to
him or, more generally, to the National Health Service as a
whole. The principal criterion relied upon is one called the
quality of life. From observation of the common fate of

children who, though very severely handicapped, have undergone the most active surgical intervention and treatment, it has been concluded that the children's lives are just not worth living. Multiple operations and the accompanying pain and distress to child, parent and nursing staff produce little improvement in the child's condition. It remains paralysed, incontinent, and often mentally disabled. Indeed, the history of treatment in England has been one of a shift away from a policy of active surgical intervention to a policy of selective treatment. Only those babies are treated who, on this criterion of the quality of their life, are worth salvaging. The others, as I suggested, usually die, as they did before active intervention was developed in the late 1950s. Indeed, it is an interesting insight into the practices of doctors in this field that, when active intervention was first introduced on a large scale, the number of still births reported to the Registrar General actually declined, suggesting that some, at least, previously included in that number were not genuine still births, but were children encouraged to die after the extent of their handicap was discovered. Also it is of interest to note that, by contrast, certain other countries, particularly Sweden, continue actively to treat a far greater proportion of babies than are treated in England, simply because the social services and institutionalised care available are so much better than in England, such that, once out of hospital, the baby's fate will not be one of distressing neglect despite the love and care of parents.

Now, let us analyse this process objectively. We must first note that the notion that there is a specific quality of life which a baby, unable to speak for itself, would not wish to have, because it falls too far below (however far that may be) what we healthy people conceive as the norm, can hardly be described as scientific. It is self-evidently an evaluation based at best on felt but unarticulated criteria. There is no mechanic's manual, no technician's guide, which indicates when treatment is justified. The doctor decides on the basis of some rough and ready calculus of the baby's future quality of life. And I use the cliché "rough and ready" because it captures the quality of the doctor's decision, a decision by rote, which has become a stereotype without need for deliberation. Furthermore, it varies with the doctor. There is no agreed course of action, even among doctors. In figurative terms, the baby in Huddersfield lives while the one in Halifax dies. Can anyone doubt that this enormously profound moral decision as to who should live and die cannot be left to doctors alone, or even to parents.

This seems so clear that you would think opposing views would be impossible. Yet, in fact, to make the point is to attract the odium and hostility of doctors in the field, who are convinced, with a sort of Messianic fervour, of the rightness of their decisions. But I persist. It is not necessarily that I disapprove of what is being done. It may be that we all, or most of us, do approve. What I find utterly objectionable is the notion that this so profound a question is rightfully for doctors alone to decide upon, so that others intrude at their peril. And it is made more objectionable by the fact that, if one is for a moment to play the lawyer, there is at least some suspicion, if not downright certainty, that the law of homicide is having its tail twisted. This would not be the first time we have decided to turn a blind eye. But we should all be given the chance to know and to decide on the basis of clearly articulated and agreed-upon ethical principles. The doctor overreaches himself in his claim for unique competence.

Nor is this ethical dilemma limited to new-born babies. It arises, for example, each time the doctor decides whether or not to try to resuscitate the person who has attempted suicide. It arises each time a doctor must decide whether a patient dying from kidney failure should receive dialysis treatment or be selected for a kidney transplant. It is an illusion to imagine that the decision will be unaffected by considerations of the 'social worth' of the patient. In the absence of any effective review of the decision, or any established principles, it will be the doctor's view which will prevail, however idiosyncratic. It arises each time the doctor weighs up what to do about his elderly patient who lies paralysed from his latest stroke and now has pneumonia. Should he treat the pneumonia, so that the patient may live another couple of weeks or months? Or should he let the pneumonia be the old man's friend, as it used to be?

Not surprisingly, such dilemmas as these have been brought before the courts in the United States. For several reasons, the courts play a far more active role in the United States than in the United Kingdom in resolving issues of this nature. Two of the most famous recent decisions have been in the Saikewicz case and the Quinlan case. In Saikewicz, Judge Liacos, in the Massachussetts Supreme Court, decided that the question whether a severely mentally retarded man of sixty-seven should receive chemo-therapy which would temporarily postpone his death from leukaemia was not one to be decided by doctors alone, but by the courts, according to principles laid down by the courts. The decision provoked screams of outrage from the medical profession. Arnold Relman, the editor of the *New England Journal of Medicine*, led the onslaught, condemning the decision as a vote of "no confidence in the medical profession". The thrust of the critics' argument was that, in the words of R. Reiss, writing in the June 1980 issue of the *Journal of Medical Ethics*, "It seems to us that the experienced physician is in a much better position to make such judg-ments than either the family or a court of law".

It seems to me, however, that there are two issues which the critics confuse. First, it must be clear beyond per-adventure that a decision such as the one involved in the Saikewicz case, though it must be made by doctors, cannot be made by reference to principles laid down only by doctors, far less the view of one doctor. It must be made by reference to socially established and institutionalised principles. The second issue is the question of who should lay down these principles. Arguably, in the United States the courts are the appropriate agency, *faute de mieux*. In

England the courts play a less prominent role and are not seen, as they are in the United States, as the great unifier in an otherwise heterogeneous country. The courts would not in my view be the proper agency to lay down the principles in England. But the first point remains intact, whether in the United States or England.

The Quinlan case is undoubtedly important for what it decided: that there comes a point beyond which a doctor is no longer under a duty to persist with forms of treatment which can be described as heroic or pointless. It is equally important because the New Jersey Supreme Court made it clear that such a decision was of such profound philosophical significance that it was for the court, representing the distillation of society's wisdom, not for doctors, to make. On these points at least, the decision was, and has been regarded as, a major advance in the development of humane and sensitive medical law.

This does not stop some, such as Lord Smith, President of the Royal Society of Medicine, arguing in the same issue of the *Journal of Medical Ethics* that "the wise and humane physician, in tune with his patient, will know very well when it is time to withdraw treatment. This decision must be made by, and the responsibility borne by, one doctor who has earned and enjoys the confidence and trust of the patient and his family. We must not allow this to become a committee matter. Still less must a decision of this kind become a matter for the courts of law. We have seen, much publicised in the Karen Ann Quinlan case, what happens when an attempt is made to invoke the legal code, and the spectacle was hardly edifying."

It may be that in England, as I have said, resort to a court may be considered less appropriate. But, on all other points, Lord Smith's view must be wrong. Such decisions simply are not to be made on the basis of a particular doctor's wisdom or humanity, great though these may be. And to denigrate the Quinlan decision is to fail to understand the splendid use of the natural law principles of freedom and privacy, as found in the U.S. Constitution. It ignores the power for good the decision has become in the United States, not only in its specific detail but also in its embracing of a notion that there is a limit to how far massive and pointless medical intervention should be tolerated.

Now consider Mrs X. She has cancer. It is decided that the cancer will not respond to treatment and that she will die within a matter of weeks or months. Given that such predictions are at best guesses, the question that then arises in the mind of her doctor is what he should tell her. Should he tell her the truth about her condition, or offer some alternative story which is perhaps more optimistic? I choose the example of cancer, as it is familiar. Of course, the questions raised are by no means limited to cancer patients. They pervade the whole range of medical care. The Royal Commission on the N.H.S. makes the point that 31 per cent of in-patients and 25 per cent of out-patients in a specially commissioned survey did not consider they were given enough information about their treatment and care.

The assumptions which underlie these questions are obvious. People do not want to die; neither do they want to know they are dying; nor could they tolerate being told they are dying; nor do they know they are dying. Some or even all of these assumptions may be well founded on occasions but they are unsupported by any evidence. They reflect the anxieties of the healthy. As Susan Sontag puts it in her book *Illness as Metaphor*, "All this lying to cancer patients is a measure of how much harder it has become in advanced industrial societies to come to terms with death." In fact, as Una MacLean shows in her paper, "Learning about Death," in the *Journal of Medical Ethics* of June 1980, what surveys there are show that the large majority of patients with, for example, cancer would prefer to know the truth. By contrast, doctors ordinarily choose not to tell.

Perhaps the most important assumption underlying the question of what to tell the patient is that it is the doctor who is uniquely qualified to decide what the patient should know. Of course, once the view is allowed that patients do not want to know the truth, rationalisations can readily be created which serve to justify this position. The notion that the patient does not wish to know soon becomes the notion that the patient should not know. One argument commonly used is that the diagnosis is uncertain. But a study by J. McIntosh published in 1978 by the Institute of Medical Sociology in Aberdeen, in the book *Relationships between Doctors and Patients*, demonstrated that uncertainty over diagnosis was not the reason for withholding information, though it was used to justify it. The better explanation for non-communication, according to McIntosh, was uncertainty not over diagnosis but over how much each patient wished to know, an uncertainty largely produced by the doctor's own anxieties. All the doctors in the study firmly believed that the great majority of patients should not be told that they had cancer, nor be given their prognosis unless it was favourable. The patients were to be given only as much information as was compatible with the retention of hope, whether justified or not. The doctors realised that some patients may indeed have wished to know the truth, but, since without asking they could not know which patients, they managed the problem by not telling anyone, unless a patient specifically demanded the truth. This may have provided the ideal coping mechanism for the doctors. But it meant that only the patient who was articulate, who insisted on the truth, and was confident enough to be persistent, got his way.

Another rationalisation resorted to is the so-called therapeutic privilege. This suggests that, as a matter of good medical practice, the doctor may withhold information from his patient if in the exercise of his discretion and judgement it would not be in the best interests of the patient's health to know. This is clearly a device created by doctors to do what is in the best interests of doctors. It may be justified on some occasions, but there is no effort to specify these occasions. Everything proceeds on the basis of the particular doctor's judgement. It all boils down to the doctor being good, gentle and kind. It would be nice if all our doctors were like this. But, just in case, can we not have some more certain guarantees that our interests, as defined by us, may be allowed to prevail? The device of the therapeutic privilege pays lip service to the principles of truth telling and self-determination, while it creates a discretionary exception which is quite capable of swallowing these principles when the doctor decides the occasion requires it.

If we look beneath these rationalisations we see an ethical principle which is certainly not part of received tradition concerning the doctor–patient relationship. The traditional view is that the doctor–patient relationship rests on trust, or at least on agreement. But what we see is an operational principle, defined by the doctor and accepted by us by default, which allows the doctor to suspend the trust, or rewrite the agreement, when in his view this is appropriate. Of course, if the patient breaks his trust or violates the agreement there may be dire consequences for him, even to the extent of his forfeiting further care. Not so for the doctor. He remains arbiter of the relationship, even to the extent of claiming the privilege of resorting to an operational principle which is the precise opposite of traditional ethics. For it is a basic moral principle of our society that we should tell the truth. If this principle is to be the subject of exceptions, and it is, of course, well recognised that there are circumstances in which it is justified to withhold the truth, or even to lie, this should only be after careful analysis and common agreement. No one is saying it is easy to tell the truth. It is a difficult, even harrowing task. It calls for the exercise of considerable skill and understanding. But the principle remains. Any exceptions clearly should not rest on the unexamined and unarticulated say-so of the doctor. Yet the practice goes on, and is defended.

The examples I have referred to so far are fairly commonplace. We would all have recognised them as typical of medical practice, even if we may not all have recognised the ethical nature of the decisions made. It may be that some of you would be content to leave things as they are, despite the far-reaching significance of such decisions. Well, let me press you a little further. Let me press the point that decisions taken by doctors are of such a nature that a check should exist on the power this decision-making grants to them. I want now to look not at specific examples but across a whole area of medical practice – that concerned with reproduction and birth. I want to identify for you the ethical principles by reference to which this area of medicine is practised. You may not as easily recognise the decisions which are made as being part of traditional doctoring. They seem far more clearly for us to make, rather than leave to the doctor alone. Perhaps, when you have heard what I suggest, you will be more prepared to accept my thesis, that doctors are involved in making decisions which are more than technical. They are ethical decisions about us. They closely affect our lives. They are made without reference to agreed principles. They invest great power in the doctor. And they are regarded, at least by doctors, as uniquely within their competence to make, such that their power is not easily checked.

So let us turn to medical practice concerned with reproduction and birth. Let me quickly suggest some of the contexts in which medicine is involved, and in which decisions are made by doctors. Obviously there is abortion. Then there is the treatment of severely handicapped newly-born babies which I have already mentioned. Then there is the screening of pregnant mothers and foetuses to identify deviations from the chosen norm. There is the provision of genetic counselling to parents, to help those who may bear a disabled child to make their decision whether or not to have a child. There is medicine aimed at inducing fertility, for example artificial insemination and, most recently, *in vitro* fertilisation, the so-called test-tube baby. And there is contraception, which includes, of course, sterilisation. On careful analysis, decisions taken by doctors in these areas of medicine, despite the superficial differences, can be shown to rest upon certain underlying common assumptions which are ethical in nature. I suggest, furthermore, that these common ethical assumptions are unstated, unarticulated and certainly unremarked, because it is probably not appreciated by doctors or lay people that they are being made. Yet, when they are identified, they can be shown to be of very great significance, reflecting and affecting as they do our approach to child–bearing, child–rearing and the value of life. You may well wish to consider who it is who should decide whether you are fit to raise children.

Consider what Professor Henry Miller of Newcastle Medical School wrote in his book *Medicine and Society*; that final decisions on such matters as planned parenthood rest often with parents, but, and I quote, "the trouble is, of course, that the parents from whom difficult decisions are most likely to be required are all too often drawn from the most feckless and irresponsible sections of the population". "The problematical issue of positive as opposed to negative eugenic policy", he goes on, ". . . is fatally complicated by the fact that, unlike the breeders of horses for courses, we don't and can't really know exactly what we want: the qualities desirable in a 1918 infantryman are not necessarily those appropriate to an astronaut." You are left in little doubt as to what should happen if we did or could know what qualities were needed!

The first assumption I would identify is that some are more fit than others for child–bearing and child–raising, with the implication that the unfit should not bear or raise children. But, if we were to attempt abstractly to devise a set of criteria of fitness to be a parent, I doubt if we would get very far. Clearly what is at the heart of the assumption is a concern for the potential child. A child just should not be born into a particular environment or to particular parents. Yet there is an extraordinary ambivalence in how this concern is demonstrated. On the one hand, it seems to be reflected in a doctor's decision to sterilise the mentally retarded girl before she can get pregnant and bear a child whose future may be less than happy. And the decision by doctors to offer artificial insemination only to stable married couples who have passed some sort of parental fitness test seems to express the same concern for the welfare of future children. Equally, Doctors Steptoe and Edwards, developers of the latest reproductive technology of *in vitro* fertilisation, have announced that they have drawn up a code of practice whereby, according to *The Times* of 14 July 1980, potential beneficiaries will have to pass the same sort of parental fitness test. Parenthood is to be encouraged, indeed facilitated, but only in certain circumstances. It is to be prevented in others. The guiding criterion is concern for future children.

But the ambivalence creeps in when a doctor with these views refuses to perform an abortion, just as much a medical practice in the area of reproduction as are the others. Where is the concern for the future child there? Or where is it when he refuses to prescribe contraceptive pills to a girl who is under sixteen? The doctor doubtless regards her as unfit to be a mother, to bring a child into the world, but his decision not to prescribe the contraceptive pills may well have precisely this effect.

In these two cases, the ethical principle of fitness to be a parent, which previously guided the doctor, seems lost, though arguably this is a situation where its application would be more than appropriate. Instead he seems to be operating on another ethical principle, that a woman ought to bear the child conceived. Whether it is in the child's best interest to be born is suddenly of less importance. It is almost as if the child is seen as punishment, that it is no more than is deserved. There is, in effect, a complicated intermingling of a whole set of principles or, some would say, prejudices or biases. On the one hand, there is a policy of eugenics, seeking the right parents. But, on the other hand, there is a policy of retribution, whereby children must be brought into the world regardless. And these policies are completely within the power of doctors to operate.

As Lesley Doyal points out in her book *The Political Economy of Health*, it is clear that in the case, for example, of abortion doctors operate a system of screening of women which has nothing at all to do with the legal requirements for abortion laid down in the Abortion Act 1967. Single women seem to be divided into "the girl who made a mistake" and "the bad girl". Women have to be very careful in their management of their relationship with their doctor. If the good girl is suitably contrite she gets her abortion. The bad girl does not. It would only encourage her to be promiscuous. Doyal quotes the remarkable conclusions of a study of Scottish doctors:

"Not unnaturally, the doctor does not like it if he and the help he can give seem to be taken for granted. The wording of her request, the wrong manner, too demanding or over-confident, even her way of walking in ('she come prancing in') may antagonise him and lessen her chances of referral. On the other hand, too passive an approach can be misinter-preted. 'You get the impression with a lot of these lassies that you could push them one way or the other and in a situation like this I tend to say keep the baby. . .' The doctors respond best to a concerned approach and tears are never amiss."

The ethics involved are crude and contradictory. Yet they pass, unstated and unchallenged, as part of the practice of reproductive medicine. We happily leave it all to the doctors and should not be surprised at the idiosyncratic and contra-dictory principles which emerge.

A second ethical assumption which underlies medical thinking and practice concerned with reproduction and birth is that a baby should not be born or, if born, should not be encouraged to live if the quality of life the child would enjoy falls below a certain standard. Of course, the first obser-vation is that what amounts to a minimum quality of life is not set out anywhere. Indeed, if one attempted to do so, the opposition and the hostility which would greet the attempt would swiftly dissuade others. Yet I am suggesting that this principle, inarticulate and idiosyncratic as it may be, is one of the most significant guiding principles in this area of medical practice. Once again, the alleged motive is concern for the child. We can see this clearly in the practice of selective treatment of severely handicapped newly-born babies. The most severely handicapped do not receive surgery or antibiotics and are encouraged to die peacefully, or, to use the words of Dr John Lorber, one of the most famous specialists, the babies are not encouraged to live. This same concern for the child is also reflected in the law and practice of abortion, where there is less than the usual opposition when abortion on the grounds that the child will be genetically severely handicapped is raised. Furthermore, the modern practice of screening pregnant mothers is posited on this assumption, that it would not be in the interests of the child if it were born genetically disabled. And we have witnessed in tandem with the enormous development of the field of genetics in the past two decades the appearance of genetic counselling.

There cannot be much doubt that in genetic counselling, too, this same assumption operates. Of course, the theory is that the mother should be given the information and then left to make up her own mind. The role of the doctor involved is allegedly that of a neutral purveyor of facts, rather than an advocate of any particular decision. I doubt if this distinction is real, since no presentation of facts is value-free, and the so-called neutral party can always, by the facts he chooses to relay and the emphasis he places upon them, manipulate effectively the decision arrived at.

Few would suggest that this ethical assumption concerning a minimum quality of life is wholly wrong or ought to be abandoned. But, quite apart from its clear lack of definition, it is important to notice the eugenic tone which underlies it. There is, perhaps, some moral danger in following a path which leads to the conclusion that the handicapped should not be born. Though we all want healthy children, health, as we know, is a term which defies

easy definition, and who is to say along what point of the
scale of handicap a baby's life would not be worth living?
Furthermore, such a pursuit of the handicap-free child
might inevitably make us less tolerant of that child who, for
whatever reason, is not caught by the screening process. Is
such a child to face a future as a freak or a reject, shunned,
because such children are just not born like that any more?
And there is again some ambivalence in medical attitude and
practice in this context. Those doctors who refuse to
perform an abortion to prevent the birth of a genetically
disabled child also claim that they are concerned only with
the child's best interests. But, to them, there is no minimum
quality to a child's life. Only in such a way, they seem to
argue, can we remain a caring society, rather than a selfish
and narcissistic one which only wants babies if they are
made in the right image. Existence is all – a view shared by
those doctors who advocate that severely handicapped
newly-born babies should be helped to live, rather than
encouraged to die. But even these doctors might perform an
abortion for a girl who had been horribly raped, or draw the
line at treating the most severely handicapped newly-born
baby. So their position also is not free from ambivalence.

These issues concerning a minimum quality of life are
profoundly difficult. What is striking is that, despite their
significance, they are not widely discussed. They are
resolved in the consulting-room and debated, if at all, in the
medical journals. But, as you have seen, the ethical assumption that there is a certain minimum quality of life is
unclear. The counter-principle, that there is no minimum
quality of life, coexists with it, again with no clear meaning
or clue as to when one, rather than the other, should operate, producing ambivalence and contradiction. Science and
technology have developed their own momentum. New
procedures such as foetal screening are introduced because
they are now possible. Any consideration of the ethical
implications is seen as quite independent and usually, if
undertaken, takes the form of capitulation before another

technological *fait accompli.*

A third ethical assumption, I suggest, is that a child has a certain worth, socially and economically, and should be conceived, or born, only if it would qualify as worth it. This is most evident in the case of abortion, when a doctor may find himself asked to certify that the birth of a child would be a detriment to the existing family's health. Here, the word "health" can be manipulated, if need be, to include the threat to the health of existing children represented by additional competition for the available resources of the family. Here the underlying concern may be, as in other cases, for the child about to be born, that he is better off not born. But there seems to be an equal concern for those children already born. Those who oppose abortion are particularly concerned at the extent to which this criterion is capable of being manipulated. It means that the decision whether a child should be born may be made to depend on the social convenience of the birth. But to argue otherwise is to say that the child should be born, even though it would not be welcome.

Despite the complexity of the argument and the conflict of principles, we can once again find doctors making decisions, giving advice, as if what was involved was a mere matter of technical expertise. Any ethical analysis which is indulged in is rudimentary at best and not exposed to wider scrutiny. Indeed, recently, doctors specialising in the field of genetics have found themselves more and more parlayed into these ethical difficulties. Through the development of foetal screening, they have been able to discover more and more about the foetus, so as to aid the parents in deciding what course to take. Now comes the problem. What if a doctor knows that Mr and Mrs X want desperately to have a baby boy? In the course of routine screening, he discovers that the foetus Mrs X is carrying is healthy, but a female. Doctors have got themselves into a considerable lather about whether or not the parents should be told this when it is likely, in our chosen hypothesis, that the mother will then seek to have the foetus aborted. The doctor may not regard the information as relevant to any decision the parents may wish to make. But, by defining what is relevant, the doctor is already making the ethical decision that only certain information should be revealed and that he should be the sole judge of this. To lie, to withhold the information, or to reveal it – each is equally repugnant to many doctors. This is, if you will, another example of the dilemmas medical technology brings in its wake. We must, it is clear, flush out these ethical problems associated with medicine at the beginning of life. They affect our future, they are ours to resolve.

So let me tie up the various threads of my argument. We have seen how decisions made by doctors are ethical in nature, calling for careful analysis. There is no evidence that such analysis is engaged in. If, for instance, you look for wise words and advice to the recently revised *Handbook of Medical Ethics* produced by the British Medical Association, you will be disappointed. For example, the section on the treatment of severely handicapped children ends in the ringing phrase, "the doctor must find a just and humane solution for the infant and the family". So far, so good; but just what is a just solution? To argue, as some doctors do, that "we learn on the job" is to support some notion of education by osmosis, or to say that they perpetuate, unconsidered, the views of their predecessors, or to admit that they receive no education at all in ethics.

We should expect not only some regularity, if not uniformity, in the decisions arrived at, but also some conformity between these decisions and those which the rest of us might make. We should also expect that doctors have some educational grounding in ethical analysis. To suggest this last crucial point is to invite scorn. "There is no room in the curriculum. We do not want to clutter up our timetable with well-meaning Sunday school exercises." My response is that much greater stress must be laid on the humanities during a doctor's training. Ethics must be a central course, taught not by some superannuated elder statesman, nor by the latest medical star in the firmament, but by an outsider, someone who is not deafened by the rhetoric of medicine. Medical schools must simply be dragged back into our world and out of their hermetically sealed cocoon of a world, in which we are counters with which the game of life is played.

The teaching of ethics would introduce future doctors to the proposition that there is the sort of tension and even contradiction between ethical principles which I have sought to demonstrate. The claim that there is only one fundamental professional ethic, "benefit and above all do no harm", would be exposed as untenable. For example, a Jehovah's Witness in danger of bleeding to death may refuse a blood transfusion, fully aware of the implications of his decision. If there were only one ethical principle in the practice of medicine and if it were solely for the doctor to dictate and interpret, it could justify the doctor in ignoring the patient's decision. But in fact, we tend to favour the ethical principle of respect for an individual's autonomy and freedom, whatever the doctor or others may wish to do. And there are other ethical principles equally strongly regarded. One very important one which should be mentioned here is the principle of doing justice within society, by, for instance, avoiding discrimination and allocating resources fairly. This is important because it suggests that the traditional notion of the doctor's obligation as being to his patient and only to his patient cannot go unchallenged. For, if justice includes the fair allocation of resources within the community, it may mean that the interests of a particular patient must properly be weighed against the larger interests of the community and that in appropriate cases the doctor should put the community first. This is the stuff of ethical analysis, exploring the tensions and conflicts between ethical principles and suggesting ways of resolving them. This is the sort of rigorous analysis to which medical students and doctors must be introduced.

Teaching ethics is not a solution, of course, although it

would represent a step forward. We must go further. The principles by reference to which doctors act must be the product of general discussion and debate. They could then be set down in some form of code of practice. There are those who oppose this or any other form of writing things down. It makes everything appear either to be black and white, they argue, or so grey that you may as well not have bothered.

There is some force in this argument, particularly when something as sensitive as caring for someone is involved. But, on balance, it is an argument I reject. The power surrendered to the doctor, the freedom and responsibility abandoned by the individual, if the appropriate principles are not laid down, are too great. They outweigh any anxieties over the problems such a code may pose. One such code of practice is at present being prepared for doctors on the care of the terminally ill, and there are others which have been prepared recently, for example the 1979 code of practice on transplantation. These new codes are badly flawed in that they have been drawn up by doctors, so perpetuating the notion that what is involved is a matter of technical expertise. But they are a beginning. We must take over. It may be that in large part we as laymen would endorse many of the decisions taken by doctors. But it is overweening hubris to deny us the opportunity to consider them first and on occasion to insist, and I repeat insist, that our views rather than theirs prevail.

5

The doors of mental illness

GEORGE says he is going to kill himself. What should we do? Should we express concern? Should we do more and, if so, what more? Is George ill? Is George mentally ill? Bill believes, quite wrongly, that the Inland Revenue is pursuing a vendetta against him. He leaves home and family and begins to wander around, living rough. What should we do? Should we try to persuade him to see someone and, if so, whom should he see? And if he says no, what then? Is Bill ill? Is Bill mentally ill? Tom believes that this country's problems will be solved only if immigrants from the new Commonwealth countries are caused to leave. He makes speeches regularly and publishes a monthly newsletter which pursues this theme. What should we do about Tom? Is he ill? Is Tom mentally ill?

These question are among the more taxing we face in our modern society. Any answers must draw on our sense of right and wrong, of propriety, of normality, of order, of law and authority, and perhaps, most significant, our sense of freedom and responsibility, especially our sense of freedom and responsibility. At what point does caring become controlling? At what point does freedom become dangerous? This, to me, is what is involved in any examination of mental illness. As I search for an answer, keep in mind that these are practical problems. Keep in mind that the easiest solution, at least superficially, is to "put people away", as the expression goes. This has a fine historical precedent. To what extent we can, or should, continue to do it is a question which will dog us throughout. Keep in mind that my concern from the outset has been with the twin notions of responsibility and power, in the context of the practice of medicine. Nowhere are these notions more clearly involved than in the context of mental illness. To be judged mentally ill is to be judged, to a greater or lesser extent, not responsible. The implications for freedom and its denial are profound. You only get your life back when others judge you responsible again.

Any consideration of mental illness must take as its starting-point the question "What is mental illness?" It is common knowledge that there are some who argue vehemently that mental illness is, in the words of the most famous polemicist, Thomas Szasz, a myth. He has it that the notion of mental illness exists as a mechanism for social control, for medicalising, medicating, even incarcerating those regarded as social misfits. It represents a conspiracy between us and the specialist, the expert. It looks respectable if the expert does it, whereas we would feel uncomfortable, or even guilty, if we used other social means to achieve the object desired. And, Szasz seems to argue, we have created a monster. The power, once granted to experts, cannot be taken away. So we stumble along and hope not too much harm is done.

Of course, Szasz does not go unanswered. Psychiatrists, psychologists, analysts and laymen line up regularly to shoot at him, each one delivering what he sees as the *coup de grâce*. They dispute the very basis of his objection to mental illness, so it is as well to recall what this is. The principal point made by Szasz is that the word "illness" is properly applied to physical illness, where a disease entity exists. No such physical disease entity exists in the case of mental illness, therefore it cannot be called illness. It is, instead, a moral or political judgement. But this argument is fundamentally flawed. The flaw does not lie in the point that there are, in fact, disease entities in the case of mental illness. Rather, the flaw lies in the failure to understand that illness, in the form of alleged physical illness, is equally a normative or judgemental term. Illness is more than the existence of a set of objective conditions. It is a judgement that a particular status, that of being ill, ought to be ascribed to someone in whom those conditions are present. Depending on the judgement made, the doctor grants or withholds the status. So there is no reason in principle why the notion of illness should be restricted to physical states. It can just as well be extended to thoughts, mood or behaviour. If it is decided that these warrant the evaluative judgement that they should be regarded as illness, then illness they can be. Equally, in principle, for want of a better term, they can be called mental illness. Thus, in short, the intellectual basis for Szasz's argument is misconceived. It is not a telling argument to say, as does Szasz, that there is no such thing as mental illness, since illness is not a thing. Despite this flaw, the insight and observations of Szasz remain valuable. He asks the right questions even if for the wrong reason. For what has to be considered is whether the judgemental term "illness" should be used in the way it is.

Before going on, perhaps I ought to respond to the arguments of those who say that there are specific disease entities and conditions, which amount to mental illness. Certainly, having accepted the notion of mental illness into our culture, you can see how our language reflects the imagery of disease. We speak of someone as "having a screw loose", of being "not quite all there", or, in American argot, of "losing his marbles". All of these are obviously mechanistic explanations. We resort to them because we do not have any persuasive non–materialist analogy to capture what we want to convey. We are after all trying to describe something which, in our heart of hearts, we suspect is a judgement on someone, that he is odd, or different, or should be treated differently, or should be avoided. There are, for example, those who regard the mind as being the product of the complex biochemistry of the brain. At least for them, the day may soon dawn when we can relate mental qualities and attributes to the brain's biochemistry. They would deduce from this the dramatic assertion that mental illness will then be shown, in fact, to be mere biochemical malfunctioning. Mental illness will then be just another form of physical illness.

Things are not so easy. This materialist way out is hopelessly flawed. Notice the circularity in the argument that mental illness is biochemical malfunctioning. It begs the question. It assumes what has to be proved: that certain particular mental states, ways of thinking, moods, behaviour, temperament, ought to be regarded as illnesses. Only when we agree that they ought to be so regarded will any biochemical abnormality be relevant. Equally, until we do agree which mental states should be regarded as illnesses, biochemistry is unimportant. For there are, of course, numerous biochemical deviations from a notional norm in all of us. Most will not be regarded as indicative of illness. Only those correlating most closely with behaviour we have already decided to categorise as mentally ill will be selected. Those who look to biochemistry, therefore, have the cart very firmly before the horse.

To those who do not sail under this flag, the mind is more than its biochemistry, though what more, and how so, is not readily clear. Denying that the mind is completely to be understood in terms of material substance, it is not readily open to them to describe mental illness in terms of diseased parts. Ultimately, they are forced to fall back on the notion of disease by analogy, as indicating a deviation from the norm which, if it were in the context of the physical body, would be called a disease. When even the notion of disease by analogy seems too strong, or causes momentary intellectual misgivings, you see the term "mental disorder" being used, conveying the notion that whatever the proper order is, or ought to be, this person's mental order is not.

So I regard the disease approach to mental illness as untenable. This is not to say that mental illness is a myth, merely that the efforts of those engaged in practising the arcane skills of mental health care to defend it on materialist grounds seem insupportable. Of course, we should note in passing that this does not seem to have threatened in any way the continued claim to recognition of mental illness. Whatever the route taken, the architects of mental illness have created an edifice, similar in size and structure to that of their colleagues in the field of physical illness. Diseases have been noted. Taxonomical skills have broken them down by genus, species, and sub-species. Specialists and sub-specialists have arisen to meet the need created by a new species or sub-species, and then, most important, people have been found who are suffering from a particular illness or disease. I have not inverted the natural course of events. I think it eminently arguable that, in the case of mental illness, the experts and categorisers came first, the people to fill the categories later, just as the buildings to house them came first. As Michel Foucault argues in his book *Madness and Civilisation*, the emptying of the lazar houses of lepers was followed by the filling of them with those who would now be called the mentally ill.

So is there a better way of understanding mental illness? The key, of course, lies in its counterpart, mental health. Just as with other notions of health, a norm is involved. In this case, it is the norm of thinking, of behaviour, mood or feeling. To describe someone as mentally ill represents a judgement that his thinking, or mentation, mood, behaviour or feeling, deviates sufficiently from the norm to warrant ascribing the status "ill" to him. And there you have the dilemma of mental illness. As a notion, it is unmanageable. If, in the case of purported physical illness, it was difficult to map out the limits and bounds of the appropriate use of the concept of illness, it is that much more difficult in the case of mental illness. Yet map them out we must. For what is at stake is a concern for each person's liberty and self-determination.

It is imperative that the power of the expert to use the label "mentally ill" not go unsupervised. But there seems no ready limit to its use, it is such a will-o-the-wisp. At least in the case of physical illness, though it is a judgemental term, it is a judgement made in the light of the presence of some physical condition. This gives some guide, albeit very rudimentary, to the proper use and meaning of the term. But the very immateriality of mental illness, its other-worldliness, its association with the subjective world of the mind, rather than any physical state, deprives us of even this guide to the limit of its proper use.

So each time we challenge the use of the term "mental illness" in a particular case there is no ready guide or boundary to point to, so as to show that the particular application of the term is inappropriate or unjustified. We are forced to challenge the very basis of the concept, to deny its validity, or to say that even if it is valid as a notion we do not think it should be applied to the particular case before us. But the entrenched power of those who manipulate the concept of mental illness and the fact that they have boot-strapped themselves into intellectual respectability serve to defeat such challenges. "If you do not believe in mental illness, what more can we say?" It may appear a weak argument, but our ready acceptance of the authority of the community of experts and their willingness, indeed desire, to use their power for their own continued existence allow it to carry the day. Equally, to say that George or Bill or Tom is not, in your opinion, mentally ill is to be met by such ready responses as "What do you know about it?" or "As experts, we think otherwise." Again the power of the expert, rather than the power of the argument, defeats the challenge. Thus, intellectually and conceptually, there are no ready limits, no rationally defensible borders, to the notion of mental illness. It is a question of accepting the whole package or being thought a fool or a rabble-rouser. The implication, of course, is that we forfeit the right and ability to question the manipulation of the notion, the propriety of its attribution to George, or Bill or Tom. All the power lies with the expert, and we must just hope and trust.

As I have said, someone is deemed mentally ill when he deviates from the appropriate norm of mental health. Let us now concentrate on this norm for a while. By so doing, I shall attempt to explain how someone comes to be categorised as mentally ill. There are, in fact, two steps. The first involves a determination that George's thoughts, or moods, are abnormal. The second entails a further judgement, the nature of which is most elusive. It has something to do with how important, and I choose a vague term at this stage, how important the abnormality is.

Consider the first step. To ask the question "What are normal thoughts?" is to expose the nature of the enterprise. Heaven alone knows what thoughts all of us harbour, or have harboured, in our time. If the norm were a composite of the thoughts and moods of all of us who confidently assert we are not mentally ill, then the norm would have no meaning, because it would embrace just about everything susceptible of being thought. So it has to be something different. It has to be a norm based on what we think people should think or feel, a standard we set for ourselves, though we may not keep it. Stated in this fashion, it can be seen that the norm involved is a moral or social or political one. It is a composite of the right moral, social and political thoughts. So as not to throw the baby out with the bathwater, I will concede that there may be near-universal agreement that certain thoughts are wrong. For example, for me to think that walking naked through the streets of London is socially appropriate would be wrong. But, even if we accept that this is wrong, there is other conduct about which there would not be near-universal agreement as to its rightness or wrongness, and, of course, near-universal agreement is only a satisfactory criterion of what is right provided you accept the principle of right by numbers. So, even at this first stage, we grant power to those claiming expertise to make moral, social or political judgements about the rightness of someone's thoughts, or mood, or feeling, or behaviour. Of course, to say that one must think right thoughts or run the risk of being labelled mentally ill is to conjure up the image of *Nineteen Eighty-Four*, or of the Soviet Union, or some other nasty place. But, unwrapped from its package of expertise, and what some have mischievously christened psychobabble, this is what you have here in your midst – more subtle, yes, and less oppressive in the fact, perhaps, but still the same.

The second step is then involved. Your thoughts are abnormal, wrong. But is the abnormality important enough to warrant invoking the judgement "mental illness"? What does "important" mean here? This is, of course, at the heart of any discussion of mental health. There are two elements in my notion of importance: that which is so threatening that it goes beyond what we are prepared to tolerate, and that which evokes a particular kind of sympathy, in that the expert involved would wish paternalistically and, perhaps, patronisingly to do something. These two elements are eminently flexible and vague, even though they are so significant. Different things threaten different people. Equally, our view of those who need and deserve help may vary with the fashions of the day. But, if the thoughts or mood or behaviour already judged to be abnormal and therefore wrong are, on these tests, also judged to be importantly wrong, then the process of segregating someone as mentally ill is set in motion. The first step is to take control over the person, because to be mentally ill is to be out of control. Usually, the very act of diagnosing him as mentally ill is sufficient to allow the expert to gain control. If any doubt arises, we are, of course, always ready to support the expert in his view. Once he is controlled, by being labelled, and thereby under the power of the expert, the question of what response should be made – what should be done with, or to, the person – can be duly considered.

The implications of this process are clear. We have chosen

to allow the coming into being of a group of people who claim an expertise in mental health, or right thinking. We have chosen to allow them to apply the status "ill" to those of our fellow men whose thoughts, or words, or behaviour, do not pass muster. We have done this knowing that the nature of the expertise is in reality the exercise of moral, social and political judgement concerning the worth of someone's thinking. We must realise that this power, once granted, is not easily taken away. But we have slept easily in our beds, secure in the knowledge that, here at least, the power is not abused. Only those whom we would all regard as having really abnormal thoughts and posing a real threat, or really in need of care, have attracted the status "mentally ill".

The reality may not conform to this cosy image. One-third of hospital beds are occupied by those categorised as mentally ill. One in eight or nine of us will, at some time in his life, be diagnosed as suffering from mental illness. Five million people in England consult their family doctors each year about their mental health. Six hundred thousand are referred to specialist psychiatric services. Twenty-one thousand are compulsorily detained each year in mental hospitals. Some have spoken of an epidemic of mental illness. Is it that the experts are being a little too zealous, seeing mental illness around every corner, spotting threatening thoughts, and people needing help with their thoughts, at every turn, or are there other explanations?

The explanation I offer is that two contradictory patterns of behaviour can be seen. On the one hand, large numbers of people seek the refuge of the status "ill". To be classified as ill is to be excused of everyday responsibility, to be treated like a child. Lacking the faith that fortified their predecessors, they turn to the new religion of mental illness, in which they may confess and hope to be absolved, as painlessly as possible, by the expert. The stigma of being categorised as mentally ill is, of course, still with us, though less pronounced. But to some it may be a price worth paying for the refuge they seek.

On the other hand, while some may choose it, others may have the status forced upon them. They, too, find the pressures of our harsh world insupportable. They are not limited to those who metaphorically crack from these pressures. They may well include, depending on the nature of the society at the time, those who do not, or will not, fit. A successful, open and confident society tolerates wide variations in thought and behaviour. A society under stress becomes less tolerant. The forces of law become more vigilant or oppressive, depending on the view taken. But the process is not limited to the forces of law. Others involved in the maintenance of the prevailing social values are pressed into aid. Mental illness experts are among them. Political differences can become deviance, a code word on occasions for illness. Social protest can become irrational and dangerous behaviour. The black man who makes a speech calling for the destruction of the "white devils" will be "remanded for a psychiatric report". Sexual predilections can become sick depravities. We begin to use madness as a metaphor for those things we disapprove of in our society. Suddenly, the metaphor takes on a life of its own. That which was metaphor now becomes illness. The doors of mental illness are cranked open to receive new classes of wrong thinkers. The expert becomes society's agent, the socialiser, even, on occasions, the thought policeman.

The similarity between the processes of criminal law and the resort to the notion of mental illness are clear, but the crucial distinction is that the criminal law does not prohibit mere thoughts, nor does it reach a verdict without trial and the right to appeal. Indeed, it is salutary to notice the interrelationship between the criminal law and mental illness. Much that is deemed immoral in our society is punished by the criminal law, but some immoral conduct is not prohibited, even though it is not necessarily approved of. The reason may be that there is sufficient disagreement about its immorality or otherwise to make the passing of legislation difficult or counterproductive.

But this is not the end of the story. There is still the possibility that, anyone engaged in, or even contemplating, this immoral conduct may be judged both wrong-thinking and a threat. If this be the case, he can always be categorised as mentally ill, and thereby dealt with just as effectively. Let me offer just one example. Consider the man who thinks about – indeed, let us go further, plans on his own – the killing of an enemy. He is guilty of no crime, even if his intentions or plans become known. Nor would he ordinarily be judged, in our society, to be mentally ill. Only if he were to carry out his plan would he be at risk, and then it would be before the criminal courts, where he could speak for himself and offer what defence he thought fitting. By contrast, consider the man who thinks of having some sort of sexual contact with a young girl, let us say aged ten, or with a young boy of the same age, and makes plans to carry this out. Should these plans or thoughts become known, he is greatly at risk of being caught in the web of mental illness. He does not have to carry out his plan, the thoughts are enough. They may not be thought to be more threatening or dangerous than those of the man with homicide on his mind. Yet one may acquire the status "mentally ill", the other not. And more, once he is diagnosed, or fixed with the label "mentally ill", his liberty and future life become something for others to dispose of, while our homicidal friend walks free.

In between these two groups are the mass of mentally ill – unhappy, awkward, social misfits, who neither volunteer themselves for mental illness nor attract the status of mentally ill because of their threatening ways. By their conduct, by their inability to cope, by their position on the outskirts of our reality, they are noticed, and it is decided that something ought to be done.

What I have sought to do so far is to demonstrate the shaky intellectual basis on which the concept of mental illness rests. It follows that very great caution must be exercised in visiting the status of mentally ill upon someone.

The implications, both in terms of the freedom and responsibility of the individual and in terms of the power of the professional, cannot be overstated. This is particularly true in those circumstances in which we go so far as to sanction the compulsory detention in hospitals of certain groups of those classified as mentally ill. You will recall that 21,000 people in England are compulsorily admitted to hospital every year. They may then be subjected to treatment without their consent, and lose most of the freedoms and rights associated with citizenship, for example voting, taking a matter to court, spending money or making a will. It is hardly surprising that the idea of compulsory detention of the mentally ill attracts the greatest concern. The grounds on which a person may be detained are set out in the 1959 Mental Health Act. They are ill defined, as befits anything concerned with mental illness. Someone may be compulsorily admitted if two medical practitioners are prepared to recommend it. In cases deemed emergencies, only one medical recommendation is needed. The person has to be suffering from a "mental disorder", which is defined, if that be the correct word, to include "mental illness", "severe subnormality", or "psychopathic personality". Then the disorder has to be "of a nature and degree which justifies detention", and it must be "in the interest of his health or safety or for the protection of others" that he should be detained. That someone's liberty should rest on such flimsy criteria, and the say-so of someone claiming expertise, is startling. But, despite numerous efforts and recommendations, the words have remained unchanged now for twenty-one years.

So it is against this background that I now turn from analysis to prescription. I offer my proposals on how we should approach mental illness in the future. I would concede, at the very outset, that there is some validity in the notion of mental illness. It offers us the opportunity to ascribe the status "ill" to someone whose thoughts or feelings, mood or behaviour, we judge to be abnormal. In granting this status we can offer relief from responsibility to the person designated ill. We can show him that we are prepared to care for him, and about him, and we can allow those who specialise in treating the mentally ill the opportunity to do so, to the extent that we judge their treatments justified. But I am acutely aware of the normative nature of the status, the difficulty of identifying the norm and the implications it carries in terms of loss of liberty and responsibility. So I would seek to define more carefully the criteria of the status "mentally ill", to limit the circumstances in which it may be applied and thus, by implication, limit the power of the expert. Obviously, I cannot do more than sketch an outline here. I offer a general framework, aware that some degree of vagueness is inevitable.

There would be three classes of person to whom the status "mentally ill" could be applied. The first class would consist of those who by their conduct, as well as their thinking, become dangerous to others. It would not be enough merely to entertain thoughts which, if carried out, would be dangerous. There would have to be some positive conduct, some action, which posed a threat to the community. In other words, there would have to be conduct which amounted to a violation of the criminal law. Care would then have to be taken to separate the criminal, who ought to be blamed and take moral responsibility, from the person who ought not to be blamed. Given that this is ultimately a moral and social decision, I see no reason why it should not be made by a committee of lay people or a jury. It is not a matter of expertise, since there are no experts possessed of greater insight into what our moral values ought to be than the rest of us. If the danger was sufficiently grave, I would condone the compulsory detention of such a person. If he were detained, there would have to be a tribunal or committee, established by law, which would periodically review whether his detention was justified. If it was not, he would, of course, be released. Such a committee or tribunal would, once again, consist of lay people, though, of course, it would hear the views of those claiming expertise. And, of course, the detained person would have all the rights appropriate to someone detained against his will, including an opportunity to appeal and access to an adviser, whether lawyer or layman.

The second class of persons would consist of those who requested help. They would be the unhappy, the depressed, those who found the stress of life difficult to bear. It would be for such a person to ask for help; help must not be forced upon him. And, if he chooses to diagnose himself as mentally ill, in that he chooses to consult those who specialise in mental health, then so be it. The usual range of services would be made available to him. There would be no case for admitting such a person to hospital unless he sought this. Is there not a risk, it may be asked, that some may choose to join this second class, so as to opt out and become free-loaders, living off the State? The answer must be that, if a person chooses to live among us but to look to the State for financial support, beyond free advice and appropriate treatment, he would have to satisfy a panel of lay people that he was unable to provide for himself. The risk of someone opting to free-load by living in a mental hospital is slim enough not to cause us concern!

The third and final class would consist of those who ought to be helped, as they appear helpless. This is, of course, a wide and potentially unmanageable category. It looks, I admit, not unlike the woolly sort of categorisation I have previously been criticising. But it need not be. It would differ in that legislation would have to be drafted which was far more carefully and narrowly drawn than the present Mental Health Act. It would differ in that helplessness would be specifically related not to bogus diseases or disorders but to demonstrable facts, which would have to be proved. Such facts would be a person's inability to perform the basic tasks of life, such as procuring food or practising hygiene or finding lodging. It would differ in that provision would be made for distinguishing between the odd, the eccentric or the apparently foolhardy and the helpless, warranting help. The distinction would turn on choice. If the person chose his way of life and did not request help, then so be it. Some may argue, of course, that the person may have chosen, but his choice was the product of confusion. This is where we came in, where caring becomes controlling, where our values as to how life should be lived are converted into normative propositions as to how others should live. If there is no evidence of choice, no indication that the state in which the person finds himself is the product of his will, then he would warrant help, if otherwise he could not sustain himself.

Some may say this makes no allowance for the person who finds himself in difficulties not out of choice but out of circumstances which he was powerless to control. I would merely remind them that we are asking here whether such a person should be regarded as mentally ill. I am suggesting he should not be. I am emphatically not suggesting he should be abandoned. But it is the job of others – whether through social services or informally in the community – to cater to his needs, and if possible to restore his dignity. To push him into the embrace of mental illness would not only achieve the opposite, it would also violate the central premise of my whole argument.

By definition, membership of this class would warrant something being done to the helpless person, paternalistic action, without his consent. It would involve compulsion and possibly detention. So provision would have to be made for a formal hearing, before any decision to impose help is made, except in the rare emergency case. Also, provision would be made for periodic review of the detention, so that no one could be forgotten, lost for ever in the back wards. It would differ from the existing situation in that I can see no reason why such decisions should be taken by those claiming expertise. Given the fact that liberty is involved, as well as a sense of caring, it is appropriate that lay people, whether as committee or jury, should decide. This would

allow us, in effect, to give substance to our claimed respect
for the Samaritan over the Levite, while ensuring that the
Samaritan does not become a Zealot or a Pharisee.

You will have noticed that in identifying these three
categories I have not referred to the various disease
categories at present used, or listed in the Mental Health
Act. As I have said, I, like many, have no faith in the
validity of these disease labels, whether it be schizophrenia,
psychopathy or personality disorder. Under the scheme I
propose, only those who come within the three classes I
have outlined would be susceptible of being described as
mentally ill. Nor have I referred to those people who may
by their conduct represent a danger to themselves rather
than to others. I take the view that if freedom and responsibility are to mean anything people must be left to choose to
destroy themselves. Otherwise you undermine their sense of
responsibility. You categorise them as mentally ill and
thereby medicalise them. Perhaps you prevent them from
killing themselves on this occasion, but only at a price, to all
of us, in terms of the inroads made into the notion of self-
determination, and, at a price to them, in terms of how they
perceive themselves and their sense of responsibility for
themselves in the future.

I am not, of course, arguing for a moment that potential
suicides or self-mutilators be ignored. I am merely suggesting
they should not be categorised as mentally ill. I would be
the first to advocate the creation of social agencies, offering
help and support, public or private. A wonderful example
of the latter is the Samaritans. But the key to the Samaritans
is that the individual has to lift the telephone himself, and,
once he calls, he is not classified as mentally ill. Both of
these are crucial in the scheme of things I contemplate.

It only remains to remind you that what I said as regards
other illnesses is equally true here. We must redirect our
energies and resources towards identifying, and then
preventing, the factors which bring about the ills I have
described. In mental illness, prevention may go to the root

of our culture. This shows us the dimensions of the task. It need not deflect us.

I began by asking you about George, Bill and Tom. You remember George plans to commit suicide, Bill feels hounded by the Inland Revenue, Tom preaches race hatred. They pose problems for us. We can resort to medicine and the arcane skills of those who practise mental health care. But what price do we pay if we do so?

6

"Let's kill all the lawyers"

IHAVE CHOSEN to take as the topic of my sixth chapter* the doctrine of consumerism. Consumerism is a form of social engineering. In the hands of government, administrative agencies, courts, and private interest groups, it can be made to serve the perceived needs of the day, to protect and promote the interests of the consumer. Ordinarily, when we think of consumerism, we think of a movement concerned with the market-place, the buying and selling of goods, making sure that the buyer does not get a pig in a poke or is not taken advantage of in ways which offend current notions of fairness.

The rhetoric of consumerism is couched in terms of consumers' rights. I am not sure that this is helpful. Appeals to rights always strike me as attempts to translate into something more substantial and worthy of respect what are in effect, merely claims or intuitions. Consumerism is better understood as being concerned with protecting what are judged, at the time, to be the legitimate interests of the consumer, in the face of the greater power of others to hurt or injure or exploit him or to undermine his power of self-

*There are six Reith Lectures and I chose Consumerism as the final one since it seemed to offer a suitable finale in the light of the previous five. Chapter 7 which follows was added subsequent to the presentation of the Lectures.

determination and responsibility for his own destiny. The aim is for a better balance of power, in the light of prevailing values.

Of course, consumerism is not limited to the marketplace. It is just as concerned with the supply of services as with goods. The consumer merely becomes the client, or patient, or whatever, rather than the shopper. For example, the Royal Commission on Legal Services, whose report appeared only recently, was set up specifically to consider the extent to which the legal profession was meeting the needs of the community. The way in which medicine is practised and organised is, therefore, equally grist for the mill of consumerism. What does consumerism have to offer in the context of the practice of medicine? You will recall that throughout my analysis of medicine I have repeatedly urged on you the need to reshape medicine so that it may better serve our needs. I have also stressed the need for us, as ordinary people, to reclaim some of the power we have chosen to surrender to medicine and medicine men. Does consumerism offer a means of reshaping medicine? Does consumerism offer a means to redress this imbalance of power? It is my contention that consumerism has much to offer. I do not present it as a panacea, nor as the only means available. Clearly, it is one approach among several. But, to me it has great potential. It is a trite observation that only if we are informed can we make responsible choices. One of the great values of consumerism is that intrinsic in it is a commitment to the dissemination of information and an invitation to the education of self and others.

There are, perhaps, three principal areas on which the attention of those advancing the claims of the consumer may focus. The first is the promotion of health. Obviously, consumerism here is very wide-ranging. It can take such forms as lobbying against cigarette advertising, seeking to ensure that cars are designed safely through the passage of appropriate safety legislation, holding inquiries into the safety of nuclear power installations, or regulating the additives which appear in our food. For the most part, action on behalf of the consumer falls to be taken by the government, since in the promotion of health or prevention of illness all of us are consumers. Equally, as we have seen, it is the government, national and local, which provides such services for preventive care and the promotion of health as health visitors or health education officers. Part of the strategy I have proposed for the improvement of our health services could well include pressure on the government, by the consumer, for the continued improvement of such services.

Occasionally, individuals, or groups, have acted as champions of certain sections of the community, or of all of us. The various organisations concerned with the elderly or the poor or with handicapped children serve as good examples. By and large, they pursue their goals through the political processes: by lobbying, by producing reports, by promoting legislation. There is no great tradition in this country of using the courts to this end. In the United States, on the other hand, the courts have been most active in advancing the consumer's interest. You will recall that it was Ralph Nader who showed the way, with his spectacular success against General Motors on behalf of the users of cars, described in his book *Unsafe at Any Speed*. One recent attempt in England was the lawsuit brought against several oil companies on behalf of some children living in Birmingham. The allegation was that the lead in petrol, which escaped into the atmosphere through car exhausts, had damaged the health of the children involved, who lived near an area notorious for the volume of traffic and the traffic congestion. The suit was lost, in the face of immense problems of evidence and proof.

It may be that the courts in the United Kingdom are unsuited to engage in this kind of wide-ranging social engineering, and that Parliament is the better place to resolve such problems. But I reach this conclusion not without regret, since, of course, parliamentary time is not as readily given over to the consideration of these issues as is perhaps necessary, given their importance. And, in the commerce of political compromise, concern for the promotion of the health of the community, through measures which rub against established interests and will show no immediate reward, becomes so much small change. It would be a salutary development for all of us if more were willing to take their claims before the courts. Our courts, although traditionally conservative and slow to move, have on occasions shown great willingness to innovate, if the cause can be shown to be just. Indeed, it was the courts who were first to champion the cause of the ordinary consumer in the market-place. Admittedly, for a variety of reasons, courts in the United Kingdom perceive their role quite differently from that adopted by many courts in the United States. Nonetheless, they have been persuaded to venture where others hesitated, and could be persuaded again. I do not suggest that resort to the courts should be the only, or even the principal, means of securing the interests of consumers anxious to promote better health. I do say, however, that it offers another possible opportunity to those whose plea for a shift in the balance of power has met with rejection elsewhere.

The second area in which consumerism may have some impact is that of medical research. Developments in the medical sciences seem to overtake us at present with such rapidity that new techniques, new medicines, new procedures, have already been adopted into medical practice before we have had any opportunity to subject them to anything approaching careful or measured consideration, far less reach any judgement. We are simply overtaken by the fact that, for example, genetic screening for a whole host of factors is now being engaged in, or by the fact that coronary-bypass surgery or heart-transplant surgery or genetic engineering are not just possibilities but realities. We, the ordinary citizens, have to all intents and purposes been overtaken, overwhelmed by such developments. We have been presented with a series of *faits accomplis*. It is not a question of whether such and such research ought to continue, or to be put into practical application. It has become a matter of how we adapt to this development. The medical scientist and technologist has won the day.

Of course, none of the developments I have mentioned, and there are countless others, is free of problems, both practical and ethical. Yet we, the consumers, are rarely heard. But it is we who are affected by these developments, whether as patients or as members of the community, the physical safety or moral integrity of which is challenged. And, if any of us should be bold, or naive, enough to raise his voice and suggest we wait a moment before opening this particular Pandora's box, the scientific establishment reacts with wounded indignation. "How dare you challenge the right to pursue knowledge, conduct research and introduce technical innovation?" There is that word "right" again. The flag of Galileo is waved in your face, as code words such as "censorship" or "standing in the way of progress" are hurled.

It seems to me that this is a very unsatisfactory state of affairs. I do not need to dwell long on the researcher's arguments, since I find them nonsensical. There has never been a time when we valued the pursuit of knowledge over all things, and this is as true in medicine as elsewhere. Let someone inject an unwanted baby with some agent, known to be toxic, but the precise effects of which are unknown, just to see what happens. He may want to know. He may even feel he has a right to know. But if he makes it as far as the jail in one piece he will certainly have a long time to ponder on the limits of this so-called right.

Clearly, we as consumers may properly assert that the values by which we wish to live simply make doing some things, or introducing some procedures, wrong. But, as I say, by and large, this process of evaluation has gone by the board. One of the principal reasons is ignorance. We do not know, or find it hard to discover, what is happening. There is no conspiracy against us. It is merely that the more technical the exercise, the more it is presumed that it is a matter for technicians to decide upon. This is true as far as the observation whether, for example, a frog which has been the object of an experiment has grown another leg. It is self-evidently not true as regards the more fundamental question, whether the researcher ought to be involved in making frogs with five legs.

There are, of course, circumstances in which reviews are undertaken of the propriety of medical scientific research or the introduction of new procedures. But, with few exceptions, such exercises are fatally flawed. Such committees of review usually consist wholly, or largely, of medical scientists themselves. Take, for example, the committee in the United Kingdom which considered in 1976 the profoundly important question of when someone shall be judged to be dead, a problem created by the development of intensive care techniques and life-support machinery. The Committee, which published its Code of Practice in the *British Medical Journal* of 13 November 1976, consisted, with two exceptions, of physicians and surgeons, some of whom were specialists in transplantation surgery. I offer no criticism of the Code of Practice, nor of the members of the committee. But the association of the Code with transplantation persuades some to reflect whether it may tend to sacrifice the interests of the moribund patient in favour of those of a potential beneficiary of his organs. My view is that the association is unfortunate, but does not, in the event, invalidate the Code. But why were there so few non-medical members, representatives of the rest of us who are not doctors, but who do not need to be to hold a view on the issue of death? Equally, in 1979 a working party set up by the D.H.S.S. published its report on antenatal screening to detect the condition called spina bifida. The technical complexities are considerable. But so too are the financial, and therefore political, the ethical and hence the moral implications. Yet the working party consisted of twelve doctors and two nurses.

It seems clear to me that better machinery must be established to monitor the progress of medical research and the introduction of new practices and procedures. We are entitled to ask, for example, what such an institutional mechanism, a review committee, for example, with a membership drawn from a cross-section of the community, would have recommended when faced with the proposal to re-start heart-transplant operations in England in 1979. In the event, two centres began to perform these operations again, without apparent reference to the views of the larger community as to the propriety of doing so, whether ethically, socially or in terms of the proper allocation of scarce resources. The Department of Health had refused to finance heart-transplant operations several years previously, but private financial support was made available. I ask what a review committee would have *recommended*, because I envisage that the various groups set up would report to the appropriate Secretary of State.

There is already in operation a good example of the sort of institutional arrangement I envisage, in the committee created to oversee developments in genetic engineering. It is called the Genetic Manipulation Advisory Group and was created in 1976. The membership naturally includes those conversant with the technical details. But it also includes, for example, trades unionists, scientists from other disciplines and lay people. To those who protest at this intrusion into the field of medical scientific research, the reply must be that only in this way can we, the consumers, for whom new procedures and practices are intended, have our voice heard before it is too late.

In the United States, developments have gone much further, particularly at the instigation of the Federal Government. The Department of Health and Human Resources has created a series of ethics committees charged with the task of overseeing research and development. There is, of course, the inevitable danger of bureaucratisation, as well as the objections already noted. By and large, however, I feel we have much to learn from how this aspect of consumerism has developed in the United States.

My third area in which consumerism has a role to play is the much more specific and more important one of the actual day-to-day practice of medicine. This is where consumerism can and should make its greatest impact. In the practice of medicine, the consumer is the patient. His interests, which consumerism seeks to assert, are those of self-determination and the power to participate responsibly in decisions made about his life. The challenge to that power comes from the doctor who, in the exercise of his professional role, threatens to infantilise his patient, to undermine his power of self-determination, to act in a paternalistic manner. Consumerism has a role to play in establishing standards which doctors must meet in their practice, in measuring the doctor's performance in the light of these standards, and in creating means of redress for the patient and sanctions against the doctors, if these standards are breached.

How can consumerism play these various roles I have outlined – setting standards, measuring performance and providing remedies or sanctions? There are several approaches. They are not mutually exclusive. We should consider each of them carefully. If all of them were implemented, it would not only be the patient who would gain. The doctor too would benefit, as would the practice of medicine.

The most obvious approach is professional self-regulation. This is an odd, paternalistic kind of consumerism, in which the professional presumes to be the sympathetic advocate of the consumers' interests. The medical profession already claims to be a self-regulating body. The General Medical Council establishes standards and seeks to ensure that they are observed. But the Council is concerned largely with etiquette, rather than competence. The various Royal Colleges, for example of Surgery or Psychiatry or General Practice, also set standards of professional competence

which must be reached before the doctor has access to
certain appointments.

That this is not enough, that more is needed, is recognised, at least tacitly, by the relatively recent establishment
in a number of hospitals of a mechanism called "peer
review". This involves a regular review and critical examination of, for example, the treatment programmes adopted
by each member of the staff. Another method of self-
regulation is the formal establishment of what is called
"professional audit". As its name suggests, doctors review
and evaluate their own and their colleagues' clinical
methods, with a view to improvement. This is an area
where there is much to be learned from experience in the
United States. In 1972 Professional Standards Review
Organisations (PSROs) were introduced by the Federal
Government to monitor the performance of doctors
working within the federally funded Medicare and Medicaid
programmes, providing care for the poor and the elderly.
Despite the initial hostility to them and the fact that they are
limited to these programmes, there is little doubt that the
PSROs are a valuable institution for safeguarding the
interests of the consumer.

But audits, as yet, are relatively uncommon. One reason is
that there are no clear guides as to the standards to be applied.
The conclusion of the Royal Commission on the N.H.S.
was that it was "not convinced that the profession generally
regards the introduction of audit or peer review of standards
of care and treatment with a proper sense of urgency".

This is something of an understatement. Adopting what
The Times of 12 July 1980 described as a "strongly defensive
attitude" at the 1980 annual representative meeting, the
British Medical Association rejected the notion of introducing medical audit. It was, according to one member,
"unnecessary, undesirable, and, in some ways, offensive".

Finally, randomised controlled trials (RCTs), so
vigorously endorsed by Professor Cochrane in his seminal
book, *Effectiveness and Efficiency: Random Reflections on Health*

Services, have, in his words, been "much neglected". Cochrane's thesis is that the effectiveness and usefulness of many forms of treatment have never been clearly demonstrated and that RCTs are of primary importance in safeguarding the interests of patients. The Royal Commission concluded that "there seems little doubt that the more widespread use of RCTs could eliminate procedures whose benefits are at present accepted simply because they have never been systematically challenged". Yet, for one reason or another, RCTs continue to be ignored.

Of course, even when it exists, professional self-regulation is always open to the criticism that it is not sufficiently energetic, that ranks will be closed to protect a fellow member, rather than opened to admit that questioning outsider. Certainly, the medical profession can never be expected to become the champion of the consumers' cause. When measures as innocuous as self-audit are met with hostile rejection, it is clear that other approaches on behalf of the consumer are called for. The profession is not going to help. Standards will have to be set and measured by others. The principle of outside scrutiny, a key feature of consumerism, seems inevitable.

One solution could be for Parliament to pass legislation on the consumer's behalf. Certainly, as regards the buying and selling of goods, Parliament has been most active. But in the context of the practice of medicine it has avoided laying down, through legislation, all but the most general guidelines within which medicine is to be practised. What Parliament has preferred to do is either leave matters to the profession or establish independent agencies, charged with advancing the interests of the patient, for example Community Health Councils or the Health Services Commissioner (the Ombudsman). The effectiveness of these agencies depends on their having terms of reference which enable them to do their jobs effectively, and on receiving appropriate co-operation from the medical profession. The attitude of doctors is crucial. If doctors perceive the agencies as adversaries, rather than partners in the pursuit of a high quality of medical care and service, then the effectiveness of the agencies is much reduced. Sadly, once again, the attitude of many doctors is one of hostility. More than most other groups, doctors have a highly developed sense of territoriality. Having fought hard to gain their professional independence, it is, of course, almost inevitable that doctors should seek to guard their achievement. Regrettably, many doctors, especially those who act as spokesmen of medical opinion, seem to translate this natural tendency into an uncritical rejection of even the slightest move towards consumerism.

Take, for example, the Community Health Councils, established in 1974. Members are appointed by local authorities, voluntary organisations and the Regional Health Authority. These councils were conceived of as bodies to represent the views of the consumer, according to the 1972 Government White Paper. They were to monitor services and inform the public. But, as the Royal Commission on the N.H.S. points out, the Councils are widely criticised by doctors as being a waste of money in hard times. As the East Hertfordshire Community Health Council submitted, in its evidence to the Royal Commission, "the system is loaded against the Community Health Council. It has little money, few staff and no sanctions, save those of public opinion." The British Medical Association, at their 1980 annual meeting, recommended their abolition, complaining that they were "interfering in matters that did not concern them". They were described as "unhelpful and disruptive". The attitude of doctors is one of "Hands off. We doctors know what is best. Just leave it to us." In this climate, it cannot be a surprise that the Community Health Councils have not produced the kind of consumer service that might have been expected of them.

Other mechanisms established by government attract the same opprobrium, and have equally been less effective than may be necessary in advancing patients' interests. For example, an established complaints procedure does exist as regards GPs. But the procedures are altogether less than satisfactory. All complaints must be made in writing to the appropriate body within eight weeks of the event complained of. The system is excessively formal, takes too much time, is too complicated, and involves complaining to the very body which administers the GP service. There is no formal statutory complaints system as regards medical care in hospitals. The Parliamentary Select Committee on the Ombudsman, in its 1977 Report, severely criticised the existing system for dealing with complaints in hospitals. The procedures were condemned as complicated, fragmented and slow. Complainants were, the Committee said, often left dissatisfied, particularly when a clinical element was involved in the case.

Clearly, if it is thought desirable that complaints should be dealt with administratively within the Health Service, the present system is in need of a thoroughgoing reform. One suggestion for reform has been to extend the powers of the Ombudsman. At present, he has a very limited jurisdiction. The great majority of complaints he receives, more than 80 per cent in 1978 for example, are held to be outside his jurisdiction. One particular limit is that he may not inquire into matters involving a doctor's clinical judgement, a phrase which is, of course, delightfully vague. So the suggestion has been made that his jurisdiction should be extended, by giving him the power to inquire into clinical matters. The Parliamentary Select Committee recommended this in 1977, as did the Royal Commission on the N.H.S. Predictably, the B.M.A. at their 1980 meeting, rejected the idea unanimously.

The picture is depressing. It may be that the interests of patients could be advanced through appropriate administrative agencies, but it is clear that the present arrangements are wholly inadequate to the task. Successive governments have been prepared to do little or nothing, until something awful attracted the attention of the press, when they deplore it as if it were not their responsibility. As the Royal Commission complained, "It is neither just nor efficient to allow one scandal after another to erupt, to institute an inquiry and then to pillory those who have drifted into the often neg- lected services." For the most part, it has been left to private charitable organisations, such as Mind or Age Concern, to champion the patients' cause. The medical profession seems bent on an unyielding policy of hostility to what it perceives as attacks on its professional integrity. For example, the Royal College of General Practitioners found that two- thirds of the GPs in a study it conducted, and these were GPs training young doctors, were unaware of patient par- ticipation groups in family practices. "Only 'That's Life' freaks*, hypochondriacs, committee types and bored house- wives would be likely to join," was the view expressed. In fact, the first group was established in 1963 and all of them had been begun by doctors.

The opposition of the medical profession seems total. As the inept *Handbook of Medical Ethics*, revised in 1980 by the B.M.A. declares, "The ideal personal doctor service . . . can exist only when the limits to it set by the state are so wide that in day-to-day practice there are no practical contraints." This sort of stubborn intransigence is unjustified, not only from an ethical point of view, particularly in a profession which claims that its relationship with patients rests on trust, and then demands to be trusted. It is also clearly out of line with the political tenor of the day. Consumerism is with us. The doctor has the choices only of accepting it willingly and co-operating, or accepting it unwillingly.

The most contentious approach to furthering the interests of patients is private litigation, suing doctors or hospital administrations or others involved in medical care. Even the mention of this raises the hackles of the medical profession. You can hear the protests forming. Nothing could be more damaging to the future of medical care than the suggestion

---

*"That's Life" is a popular television programme concerned with consumerism.

that patients sue their doctors. But, if you accept that the power and freedom of the patient are in need of protection, you have already seen that existing ways of achieving this protection are less than outstanding successes. Self-help, in the form of litigation, may then warrant careful consideration. My view is that it does have some role to play, though rather a limited one, in establishing standards of practice and ensuring that they are met.

Of course, mention litigation – suing doctors – and most people will immediately think of the United States. Indeed, one of the problems which bedevils any examination of this aspect of consumerism is the passion it engenders. And this passion is largely the product of unthinking and misinformed allusions to conditions in the United States. So we have to tread slowly and carefully. We have to navigate in an area in which a poster such as "Support a lawyer. Send your child to medical school" is one of the milder forms of comment from the medical profession.

Let us consider some examples of consumerism through litigation, in the context of medical practice. The first example is a highly charged topic, known in the United States as the doctrine of informed consent. This has not gained much ground yet in the United Kingdom. It is the product wholly of courts, of case-law not statute law, and represents the courts' response to what is seen as an unmet need. The doctrine of informed consent, simply stated, has it that a doctor has an obligation in law to obtain the consent of his patient before embarking on any procedure. But it goes much further than that, as can be seen, for instance, in the famous California case of *Cobbs* v. *Grant*, decided in 1972. For it also requires doctors to advise their patients of all material risks involved in the proposed procedure, so that the patient may make an informed decision on what course to take. Clearly, this is a classic exercise in consumerism. The patient is the consumer, utterly dependent on the professional, and therefore given a right of redress if he is subsequently harmed. As a doctrine, informed consent flies the flag of self-determination against the otherwise ever-present paternalism of the doctor.

For years, doctors have responded to patients' questions with answers such as "Don't worry about that" or "Leave it to me". They have even persuaded patients to agree that the doctor, in performing any procedure or operation, may do whatever he thinks is necessary. For example, women have had breasts removed without being consulted, after biopsy has shown the presence of a tumour, or have undergone a regime of hormone treatment ignorant of and therefore unprepared for some of the effects it has produced. Consumerism is designed, here, to protect the interests of the consumer, the patient, by requiring that the final decision as to what shall be done to his body rests with him and not with the doctor. And, of course, it has been reviled by a large sector of the medical profession, as interfering in, and thereby damaging, the delicate relationship between doctor and patient. As I have said, it is a doctrine far more highly developed in the United States. Doctors and lawyers in the United Kingdom seem to delight in ridiculing it and preaching strongly against any movement towards it. The ridicule is, in my view, unwarranted and born largely of the sort of chauvinistic and lofty ignorance which the English have developed into a higher art form. Of course, there are examples of unjustified litigation, of unscrupulous patients and lawyers and excessive awards of damages. But these are the exception.

There is little doubt that consumerism, in the form of the doctrine of informed consent, promises to transform the doctor–patient relationship. It reasserts the notion that the patient is a partner in any enterprise concerning his health and cannot be a partner if he is kept in ignorance. Just as important, the patient owes it to himself to take responsibility for himself, thereby redressing the balance of power between him and the doctor. That the doctrine had to be developed by courts may be unfortunate to some, but it had to be developed by them simply because there was no other agency willing or able to do so.

The doctrine of informed consent as it is now operated in the United States has undergone a considerable development from its original premise. Here is where misunderstanding comes in. The courts have expanded the doctrine. Patients suffering unexpected harm have sued their doctors and been successful, even in circumstances where, in the view of most, the doctors have not been at fault, where they have done all that could have been expected of them. Take the case of an otherwise healthy woman about to undergo an operation for a leg injury, caused by jogging. The surgeon visits her and explains in general terms what the operation involves. He does not mention – who would? – that there have been two reported cases in the literature of complications following this operation. After all, the operation has been performed many hundreds of times. Her operation becomes the third to be followed by complications. She sues her surgeon, claiming she did not consent to the operation because she was not informed. This is what makes doctors furious. The doctor has done all he can, all that anyone would expect, yet the patient, because she now, unexpectedly, has unsightly scars or a limp, is seeking money by suing him.

The explanation is not hard to find. There is no well developed health service, of the kind we in England have, in the United States. The old and very poor get health care, of a sort, free of charge. The rest depend on their insurance cover, which often is inadequate, or on savings. Other social welfare benefits of the range provided here are also less available. Thus, if someone suffers harm unexpectedly, he needs money to pay for additional medical care or to meet other costs. With no one else to look to, the best source of money is the insurance carried by the doctor. The patient has made some small contribution to this when he paid his fee to the doctor and, after all, it is not the doctor who will pay, it is his insurer. The doctor will pass on the costs of his insurance premium by spreading them among his patients in the fees he collects. To get this money, however, the patient must sue the doctor and the doctor must be found liable. And, in holding him liable, it appears that the court is saying that he did something wrong, he failed to obtain informed consent. In truth, the court is merely ensuring that some form of social welfare system operates, paid out by insurance and funded from patients' fees. It has to do it by the sleight of hand of judging doctors to be at fault and therefore liable to their patients. Perhaps it would be more honest if the courts said that doctors should be liable regardless of any question of their fault. This is, in fact, the effect of their decisions, even though they are expressed in terms of a failure by the doctor to obtain informed consent. The object of the exercise is, after all, to compensate where compensation is needed, and the doctor's insurance is the best source available. But the American courts have as yet been reluctant to go so far as to endorse openly liability without fault, perhaps for fear that, if they were so honest, the powerful lobby of the medical establishment might persuade the Legislatures to take action to limit by statute the courts' power in this area.

A system of adequate health care, free of charge, and an adequate welfare system would, of course, obviate the need for this form of consumerism, at least as a device for compensating patients who have suffered harm. But in the United States they do not exist. Until they do, using the doctor's insurance to pay for patients' needs is as good a solution as any. Clearly, there are numerous disadvantages. As insurance premiums go up to meet claims, so must the doctor's fees go up, so that some would-be patients are priced out of the market. There are some unjustified claims. Doctors are persuaded to practise defensive medicine in the vain hope of avoiding liability. And, finally, some of the openness in the relationship with the patient has been eroded (rather than enhanced) in that doctors have resorted to hiding behind carefully drafted consent forms instead of talking to their patients.

In the United Kingdom, on the other hand, there is still a social welfare system and free health care, at least for the moment, which can serve as the basic source of funds for patients who complain of harm. So there is obviously less need in the United Kingdom for this form of consumerist litigation, so common in the United States, in which money is the sole objective. But consumerism is not concerned only with procuring money compensation when harm is suffered. It is concerned as much with establishing the principle of respect for the patient's legitimate interests, one of which is his power of self-determination. So it may be that litigation, or the threat of litigation, *is* needed here, in circumstances in which the protection of a principle, the patient's self-determination, is the objective. Furthermore, given the profession's reluctance to discipline its members, litigation could well provide the necessary sanction, or impetus, to ensure that proper standards are observed. I would not regard it as a bad thing if more lawsuits were brought against doctors or hospitals in, for example, cases in which a patient in a mental hospital was treated without consent, or in a case in which the full implications of a particular form of treatment were not explained to the patient, or were discussed only with relatives or the patient's spouse. Such actions would, in my view, lead to a healthier respect for the patient's interests and responsibilities than at present seems to exist. And they would tend to ensure that standards of practice were established which met the approval of outsiders, and were adhered to.

An even more widespread form of consumer litigation in the United States is the action for negligence in circumstances other than the failure to obtain informed consent. The patient claims that he has suffered harm because of the failure of the doctor or hospital to behave in a way which could reasonably have been expected of them. Although the number of cases brought each year in the U.K. is rising, it is still a very small number, many, many times smaller than the number in the United States. The reasons are complex.

There are cultural differences, in that, unlike the English, the American is more willing to have recourse to the courts, and less willing to accept what he may see as second best, since he is paying for it. There are differences born of the greater resort to surgery in the United States than in the United Kingdom. Surgery carries greater risk of harm than less invasive forms of therapy, but in the United States it produces higher fees, which doctors have come to regard as their due. Indeed, in more general terms, it is fair to say that doctors in the United States have tended to abandon primary care in favour of high-cost specialities. And with the growth of specialisation comes the lack of development of any close relationship with the doctor, which is another explanation for a greater willingness to resort to litigation.

But by far the most important difference is that, once again, the patient in the United Kingdom has less incentive to sue, because he has less need of the money which success in the lawsuit would bring. Once again, the English patient needing further care or disabled in any way can look initially to the Health Service and social security. His American counterpart can expect less, so must get the money he needs through the informal and expensive social security system of the doctor's insurance. Despite publicity to the contrary, the sums awarded in the United States will not be great. On average, a successful claimant can expect about £5,000 to £10,000 which, given the cost of further health care for example, is not high. So, when the need of the patient is for money compensation for harm suffered, consumerism through the action for negligence fills a need in the United States which is already largely met in the United Kingdom.

But consumerism may have two additional goals. The first is to provide money, when the state system does not provide enough. The second is to ensure that the doctor observes standards which respect the interests of the patient. Can the action for negligence achieve either of these? First, take the case in which a patient is harmed, for whatever reason, and is in need of money to purchase care over and above that available from existing social security sources.

You will recall the case in Birmingham, the case of *Whitehouse* v *Jordan*,* in December 1979. The Court of Appeal threw out a judgement for £100,000 awarded to a little boy who suffered severe brain damage at birth. Amid all the trumpeting over the vindication of the doctor, people seemed to lose sight of the realities of the case. This was one of those cases in which a large amount of money was needed to pay for care which was called for, beyond what was forthcoming from the State. The question really before the court was, simply, who should pay. One option was the little boy's parents. This would mean that he would get nothing, as they had no money. It would mean that his mother would struggle on, as she had done for the ten long years before the case even reached the Court of Appeal. Another option was the doctor. The court would have had to decide that the doctor was negligent. Sometimes doctors are incompetent. But this is not often the case. The Court of Appeal in the Birmingham case decided that the doctor had behaved reasonably and competently. The court could still, however, have decided that he was negligent. But, you say, this sounds contradictory, that the court first decides the doctor has done nothing wrong and then decides he was negligent. It need not be contradictory. It would merely involve redefining the concept of negligence. In common speech, negligence may well still mean carelessness. But its legal meaning need not be the same. Take the words insanity or duress. Their meaning in terms of law is quite different from the meaning they have in common speech.

After all, negligence is merely a legal device. It is flexible. Its meaning is not set in stone for ever. It, like the whole of the law, is dynamic. Just as social circumstances and social needs change, so must the law change and adapt. Negligence is a legal tool doing a job. If the job changes, the tool can be reshaped. It could have given the court the chance to develop the law, so as to give the little boy the money he

*I should mention that it was a namesake, not I, who was counsel for Jordan.

needed. The court could have decided that, even in the *absence* of fault on the part of the doctor, he *was negligent*, by redefining negligence. This, in the view of many, is what has happened in the United States. Negligence there has lost much of its quality of blameworthiness or fault. Of course, doctors who are found negligent get hopping mad. They have not been negligent, they argue, meaning they have not done anything wrong. They do not understand, because it is not made clear to them, that negligence is no more than a legal device allowing a particular socially desirable conclusion to be arrived at. It has become a convenient device whereby needed money can be channelled to those who have become the casualties of modern medicine.

But why, you ask, do the courts have to talk of negligence at all, since it does inevitably carry that tag of carelessness which inevitably harms a doctor's reputation? Why do the courts not just create a new legal device to achieve the desired result? Well, traditionally, courts, particularly in the United Kingdom, are reluctant to break entirely fresh ground. They are not like Haroun al Rashid sitting under a palm tree, dispensing justice. They tend towards conservatism. They prefer to move slowly, gradually, so as not to take the world by surprise. Some innovations, they think, are better left to Parliament. Of course, the precise calculation of what is for Parliament and what for them varies with time, the particular judges, and whether or nor Parliament chooses to do something. The fact that courts in the United States feel less inhibited is one reason why consumerism through litigation is so much more developed there.

In the Birmingham case, the Court of Appeal decided that the doctor was not negligent. All this means is that the court resisted the invitation to extend the legal meaning of negligence, whatever its meaning in common speech, so as to allow the little boy to recover compensation from the doctor. The court was right to do so,* not because of any

*The House of Lords affirmed the Court of Appeal's decision in December 1980 but has not at the time of writing given its reasons.

question whether the doctor was at fault or not. This can be irrelevant, as we have seen, if the goal of compensating the boy is deemed socially desirable. The real reason is that if doctors were held liable, it would be their insurance which would meet the cost. But the insurance premiums paid by doctors in the United Kingdom are insufficient to meet such claims on any scale. Nor could doctors easily pay increased premiums since, within the N.H.S., they could not pass on the cost of such increases to patients by way of increased fees. Thus, neither party to the litigation in Birmingham ought to bear the costs of the care the little boy needed, despite the fact that we may agree he should receive it. The result was that he got nothing.

But what of the case in which the doctor was negligent, was incompetent? As I have said, this does not happen very often. But imagine it did, and money compensation beyond what the existing state system provides was needed. Does negligence litigation have a place in such a case. At present, of course, it does in the few cases in which it arises. Some argue that it should continue to do so. It keeps doctors on their toes, it is said, and probably their insurance could cover the cost. It may well be that the threat of negligence litigation is one factor which keeps doctors up to the mark. But it means that, at present, the person injured through negligence is compensated. The child who cannot show negligence gets nothing, though he may have suffered the same injury. The negligence system is concerned with how the injury is caused, rather than the fact that it has been caused. I am thus led to the view that it is necessary to separate the needs of an injured party for compensation from the need to ensure that the doctor observes certain standards of ethical behaviour and of competence.

This leads me to the third option for meeting the financial needs of the little boy and any other injured party. A fund could be created, managed by an appropriate government agency and financed from public revenue. Money would be provided as a matter of course, on proof of need. In my view this is clearly the only proper solution. There is a precedent for it in the case of the children damaged by whooping-cough vaccine, although in this case the numbers involved were admittedly small. But, only recently, in 1978, the Royal Commission on Compensation for Personal Injury rejected this view. The reason given was, inevitably, cost. But the cost arguments are not so convincing. The compensation awarded could be less than at present awarded by courts; for example, damages for pain and suffering could be eliminated. The costs now reflected in lawyers' fees and insurance costs and premiums would be saved. And novel ways of financing such a fund could be found, if the will were there. Once again, we are dealing with the need for government to make a political choice. Funds have been found for other social programmes of arguably less merit. I submit that the matter deserves reconsideration. Lord Justice Lawton echoed this view when he concluded his judgment in *Whitehouse* v. *Jordan* in the Court of Appeal by saying that "the victims of medical mishaps of the present kind should be cared for by the community, not by the hazards of litigation".

So this would mean that, for the purposes of providing compensation, consumerist litigation through the mechanism of negligence, so much a feature of American consumerism, has no place in the United Kingdom. But does it have a place so as to enforce standards and ensure competence? In my view it does not. The incompetent doctor does not pay any damages awarded against him if someone is harmed. His insurance company does. He is not disciplined by his professional body, so that others might not be harmed, since the General Medical Council chooses not to take jurisdiction in matters of competence. And the resort to negligence actions on any scale may well drive doctors into defensive medicine. Furthermore, it is quite inappropriate to leave the establishment of general standards of conduct and the means of securing that they are observed to the whims of private litigation and to the lottery such litigation often proves to be. This does not mean, of course, that the consumer should not be protected from the incompetent doctor, nor that all doctors, competent or otherwise, should not be subject to review and assessment. But litigation is not the proper way.

Consumerism must take another tack. A wholly new system of supervision and sanction must be created, with the power to suspend the incompetent or even remove from practice those found to merit it, whether on grounds of incompetence or ethical impropriety. It could take the form of a tribunal or committee of review. The impetus will have to come from the consumer and the consumer will have to be prominently represented on any tribunal or committee which is set up. Other professions or groups are slowly coming to realise the importance of this approach. The legal profession, for example, is edging towards this solution and the idea of an independent review body to police the police is the focus of much debate. Whether such a body should be created under the auspices of a government department or should be independently constituted, and who should appoint its members, are matters of detail to settle once the principle is accepted. Clearly, if the jurisdiction of the Ombudsman were extended, as I suggested earlier, half the problem would be solved, since in the Ombudsman we have an established and respected institutional mechanism. But the role of the Ombudsman is largely admonitory. So as to achieve the purposes I outline, he would have to be given power to take remedial action of the sort I have mentioned.

Solving this problem is a task which consumerism has only just begun to grapple with. It is very much a task for the future.

7

The last taboo

IN this final chapter I want to pursue at greater length three issues I have already touched on: they are the role of technology in medicine and the not unrelated topics of the care of the dying and the determination of death. Let me take technology first. It warrants more consideration here because nothing epitomises more obviously the challenge which medicine in the future faces. Resort to medical technology of ever greater complexity may have some rewards for us. But it also typifies what I have suggested is the wrong approach to the provision of medical care and the promotion of health. The question before us is how to identify and then maintain the proper balance between the good and the undesirable.

Perhaps I ought to explain that when I use the word "technology" I have in mind the development and use of tools and machines, and the mechanical skills that go with them. Although I do not discount medicines, since they are tools, my attention will be focused primarily on mechanical tools. Some examples are the X-ray machine, the hypodermic syringe, the blood-pressure gauge and the scalpel. These have all been with us for some time. They are now deemed so necessary a part of our daily lives that to question their use would be regarded as absurd, a view I do not challenge here. Then there is the respirator, the kidney dialysis machine, the C.A.T. scanner, which can sketch at a cost of £450,000 *per* machine a picture of the brain or other soft tissue, and the pathology laboratory's array of diagnostic equipment, complete with the latest computer. These are examples of the more recent technical paraphernalia which now are part of the armamentarium of modern medicine. It is these I shall concentrate upon. I do not think it could be said that these modern advances are different in kind from their more well-established predecessors, such as the ones I have listed. Furthermore, it may be that these predecessors in their time posed ethical questions of the kind I wish to raise. My suspicion, however, is that the ethical questions now raised by technological developments are more profoundly challenging than has ever been the case in the past, and so warrant treating modern technological innovations in medicine as qualitatively different from what has gone before.

One point must be clear. There is little point in bemoaning, regretting or criticising what has come to pass. There are those who regret the development of, for example, the motor car or nuclear fission. Equally, we may wish to weigh up the pros and cons and say, on balance, that we would be better off without being able to fertilise human ova in a Petri dish (the so-called test-tube baby), know the sex of a foetus long before it is due to be born, or keep the irretrievably unconscious patient in a state of suspended animation for weeks and months on end. But this is a pointless exercise. These innovations are all with us and no amount of wishful thinking will make them go away. The only fruitful exercise is to ask how what we have should be used. In this way we may regulate the future, on the lesson of the past, so as to avoid the dilemmas we now face. Even this sort of measured response and evaluation is not easy. For, as I have suggested, developments in science and technology tend to acquire a momentum of their own, such that they pass beyond ready control. Once the genie is out

of the bottle, it is not a question of putting it back. That is
already impossible. It is a question of making sure it does
your bidding, rather than your doing its.

I have already referred to the irritating and singularly ill
conceived argument of some scientists and engineers – that
they are neutral researchers, seekers after knowledge. Their
motives are solely concerned with truth, they argue. They
cannot be held responsible for the mess mortals make of
their innovations. It is always the politicians and others who
are responsible for the ills which later transpire. I say this is
an ill conceived argument, despite the tenacity with which it
is held by the scientific establishment, for several reasons.
First, a scientist is not neutral; he lives in our world and his
responsibilities are to our world. He cannot detach his
normative self, the part of him which makes judgements
and evaluates things, from that part which conducts experi-
ments. By pursuing research he is already making several
value statements, for example that he ought to pursue
research, that he ought to be allowed to pursue research,
that the pursuit of research is a good thing and that the
pursuit of this particular research is a good thing. Second,
the assumption that knowledge and truth are some sort of
ultimate deities, the worship of which guarantees a lasting
state of grace in the worshipper, cannot go without
challenge. There are countless examples where knowledge
and truth are not pursued because the pursuit would
challenge values we hold more dear than them. In other
words, knowledge and truth as conceived of by the scientist
are not necessarily, or always, the ultimate values in our
society. Take for example someone who wished to carry
out an experiment which was potentially life-threatening.
Would we countenance his experimenting on, for example,
prisoners, or consenting participants, or even, if we had
them, killers condemned to die? The answer is that we, or
most of us, would not. Certain values we will not compromise with, even if the cry is heard that this is standing in
the way of the pursuit of knowledge. Indeed, to choose an

albeit extreme example, Karl Brandt, who was responsible
for much of the human experimentation which took place in
the concentration camps, was hanged after the Second
World War because he chose not to observe these first
principles in his pursuit of knowledge.

Despite the strength of such arguments against the
simplistic notion of the value-free scientist and engineer
who should be left to pursue knowledge and technical
innovation, the pursuit goes on. Of course, it is not
unbridled and limitations are set as to what ought to be
done. To that extent scientists speak out of the other corner
of their mouths, and point to the ethical codes under which
they work, notwithstanding that theirs is a value-free
exercise. But, of course, if an outsider, a non-scientist,
concerns himself with such ethical codes, he is quickly
reminded that he is trespassing on the scientists' preserve.
This involves an argument which changes sides half-way
along, for if matters of ethics are involved it is open for all
to comment. Thus, the momentum of scientific and technological development which I spoke of persists and is
extremely difficult to check without attracting the universal
odium of the scientific establishment. And this is as true in
medicine as in other areas. For example, the continued
pursuit of more and more complicated diagnostic tools goes
on as if in a vacuum, insulated from questions such as
whether the growing expense justifies the exercise, or
whether being able to identify certain physical phenomena is
particularly worthwhile if once they are identified little can
be done but to tag with the appropriate label.

There has appeared in medicine the well-known pheno-
menon which I have called the technological imperative — if
you can do it, you ought to do it. Thus, the mere existence
of equipment dictates that it be used. As we have seen, this
is attractive to the doctor trained to think of himself as the
problem solver and scientist. Furthermore, it serves to
justify the purchase of the equipment. If you have recently
fitted out a modern intensive care unit, you will want to use

it, both to prove how essential it was and because not to use it may now be thought to be neglect of the patient. You see the cycle developing momentum. The innovator develops the equipment, the producer needs to sell it, so appeals to the latent engineer or scientist in the doctor. The doctor recommends it be acquired and once it is acquired feels compelled to use it. That it may not have been necessary, that it serves to perpetuate an unfortunate model of medicine and the pursuit of health, that it attracts resources away from areas where greater benefit to health may be achieved, that patients do not seem to gain a great deal from it, that operational errors are made – all these and more are lost in the technological imperative.

How should we respond to this? First, we must notice that there are two important factors to be weighed in considering technological innovation in medicine. They are the implications, first, in terms of resources expended, and, second, in terms of ethical problems posed. I do not wish to dwell here on resources, but given the finite amount of money and manpower available for health care it is clear that some analysis in terms of costs and benefits is called for. These analyses, however, are notoriously hard to carry out. It is not easy to demonstrate that spending £x to treat 1,000 patients a year whereby 150 have their life expectancy considerably increased is less justified than spending it on putting fluoride in drinking water so that the incidence of dental caries is drastically reduced, or less justified than spending the same amount of money in wiping out the waiting-list for hernia operations so that working men may return to work. The problem becomes even more difficult when one recalls that any analysis must be seen in the light of the changing fads and fashions of medicine, whereby a particular innovation is first greeted enthusiastically and then later challenged or abandoned, such as the transplantation of such organs as the liver or lungs or even the heart or the massive care devoted to all babies born with spina bifida. Further, such analysis must take account of the politics of medicine, whereby the consultant in the teaching hospital has his hands on more levers of power than do others. Certainly, such cost-benefit analyses must be carried out despite their difficulty. A considerable number of studies have already been undertaken, particularly in the United States, though the field is relatively new as a rigorous exercise rather than a hit-and-miss affair. Unfortunately, many of the studies are flawed. Most, for example, have been carried out by economists who, perhaps, lack the necessary training and insight to take account of the competing moral and spiritual values involved. Their work, therefore, is at best a partial guide and leaves unanswered the various ethical problems which call for resolution. Gavin Mooney, Director of the Health Economics Research Unit at Aberdeen University stoutly defends cost-benefit analyses in the December 1980 issue of the *Journal of Medical Ethics*. They are, he concedes, separate from any consideration of medical ethics, but they can reveal inefficiencies and irrationalities of policies directed towards certain goals. One difficulty with such an argument is that efficiency, consistency, or rationality are in themselves ethical principles which may not always be acceptable if in the pursuit of them other values deemed more worthwhile are ignored. Other cost-benefit analyses have been undertaken by those with axes to grind, so that the results tend to be self-serving. For how you value a life or a limb or a limp may well be a product of the particular proposal you are making, since it is hard to argue that they have any constant and objective value. As Guido Calabresi, an American lawyer, has pointed out, we make rather curious social decisions concerning risks. For example, we may choose not to install a traffic light at an intersection despite the relatively low cost and the annual two or three deaths at the intersection caused by colliding cars. We may, on the other hand, choose to spend large sums, relatively speaking, to search for and rescue some mountain climber who has been fool enough to go climbing in a blizzard.

J. A. Muir Gray makes the point well be referring to the 1978 study conducted by the Office of Health Economics. Under the heading of "Values of life inferred from several public policy decisions", he cites the following table, drawn from the study:

Decision	Implied value of life	Comment and source
Not to introduce child-proof drug containers	£1,000 maximum	In 1971 the Government decided not to proceed with the child-proofing of drug containers.
Legislation on tractor cabs	£100,000 minimum	In 1969 the fitting of cabs to farm tractors, to reduce mortality risk to drivers was made compulsory. The cost per annum was estimated at £4 million (£40 for each of 100,000 tractors). About 40 lives would be saved annually.
Changes in building regulations as a result of partial collapse of Ronan Point high-rise flats	£20,000,000 minimum or perhaps actual	After a high-rise block of flats partially collapsed, killing some residents, the report of the inquiry recommended changes in the building standards of such blocks. It has been estimated from the change in risk and the costs involved that the implied value of life was £20 million.

Not to provide treatment for chronic renal failure for a person aged 50	£30,000 (Office of Health Economics estimate 1976–7 prices)	Particularly in regions where facilities are in short supply, a person over the age of 45 or 50 may stand little chance of being accepted for treatment by dialysis or transplantation.

Clearly, there is much to be done here before we can make intelligent choices based on an understanding of the implications, in terms of resources, of the development and introduction of medical technology.

Now let me turn to the ethical implications. There cannot be any doubt that very many of the ethical problems which bedevil modern medicine can be traced to technological developments. Take the example of kidney dialysis. About 2,000 people each year in the United Kingdom fall victim to kidney failure. Access to a dialysis machine means life to those whose kidneys fail, but calls for the awful and awesome decision as to who is to receive the benefit of a machine, when demand outstrips supply. In a parliamentary reply on 2 June 1980, the Secretary of State told Parliament that about 1,100 people were able to begin dialysis in 1978, an increase from 600 in 1971. But despite an increase in the number of successful kidney transplant operations performed, this still means that hundreds will still die each year from kidney failure. The question arises of how many machines ought to be made available when they cost about £6,000 to buy and between £8,000 and £12,000 each year to operate. Furthermore, the difficult question arises as to what the proper relationship between dialysis and transplants should be. Should a patient whose transplant fails automatically have access again to a dialysis machine? These are just a few of the ethical problems related to dialysis, there are many others.

The recital of ethical problems is equally long and

complex when other technological innovations are considered. There is, for example, the mass screening of women for breast cancer. The screening may itself be harmful. Furthermore, the discovery of the tumour may not significantly affect the mortality of the woman, although it may on occasions increase the sum of her unhappiness by causing her to know that much earlier. There is the elaborate technology of life support which has served to reinforce our unwillingness to admit death. There is transplant surgery. A question concerning the transplanting of vital organs which still awaits an answer is whether it is justified in terms of the results produced, leaving aside any consideration of cost. Equally difficult is the question of the circumstances under which organs may be removed, whether from the dead or the living. For example, should the law in the United Kingdom be changed to allow in the case of organs removed from the dead for the routine salvaging of viable organs without the need for consent of anyone, unless the dead person had registered an objection during his lifetime. This is the solution I advocate as long as we continue to endorse such surgery. It would favour the interests of those who may otherwise die. But it would do so only at the cost of ignoring the strongly held views of some who believe a corpse should be inviolate, and express concern that a person may not, for whatever reason, have registered an objection, yet may be opposed to his body being used for transplant purposes. The feelings of relatives of a deceased person could also be deeply hurt if organs from his body were removed without their knowledge or leave.

The problems are no more simple in the case of donations of organs by the living. Obviously the first point is that a living person may not donate an organ vital to his continued existence, such as his heart. This is not an idle point since examples exist of parents or relatives or even strangers offering vital organs for transplant. An early example reported in *The Times* of 20 August 1968 was of volunteers prepared to offer their hearts for transplant into ex-President

Eisenhower who was at that point near to death. Some would argue that donations of major organs (clearly blood in appropriate measure presents no problems) by the living should never be countenanced, despite the apparent consent of the donor, because such consent can never really be valid. The donor is usually a close relative of the patient. Under such circumstances, the pressure conscious or unconscious applied by family, friends or even the patient make any notion of voluntariness unrealistic. The donor may indeed later feel bitter or resentful at having been put in a situation in which he felt he had no choice. And the issue of consent is particularly difficult in the case of children. Should the parents of a ten-year-old child be allowed to consent on his behalf to his donating a kidney to his young brother? I find myself unable to support the argument that such a consent is valid. Ordinarily, the law stipulates that parents may only consent to that which is in the particular child's best interests. Courts in the United States, particularly in the unreported cases in Massachussetts which preceded the first kidney transplants in 1954, have persuaded themselves that the removal of a healthy kidney from a healthy child may indeed be in the child's best interests. The reason offered is that the child will feel benefit psychologically from knowing that he has saved his brother, whereas he would otherwise be grief-stricken. The high point of this reasoning can be found in the Kentucky case of *Strunk* v. *Strunk*, (445 S.W. 2d 145, 1969) in which the court allowed the removal of a kidney from a 27 year old with an alleged mental age of six for transplant into his 26-year-old brother on the ground that the donor "was greatly dependant on [his brother] emotionally and psychologically and that his well-being would be jeopardised more severely by the loss of his brother than the removal of his kidney". I find this reasoning most unpersuasive. I take the view that until a child reaches an age at which he may make an informed and mature decision for himself, surgery of this kind should not be performed. Finally, there is the tightrope walk of chemotherapy, used to treat tumours, where the line between killing the patient and killing a part of him is so narrow that Senator Hubert Humphrey was moved to describe his treatment for cancer of the bladder, from which he eventually died, as "chemical death".

I could go on. All these are agonisingly difficult ethical dilemmas, but it is another unfortunate and disquieting consequence of their arising out of the practice of advanced technology medicine that, because they are a consequence of the use of technical measures, they are treated as questions for the technical expert, the doctor, to decide. They are another species of the ethical question treated as a medical matter and therefore properly for the doctor alone to decide which I examined earlier. Once again it is obvious that this view cannot be sustained. A doctor has no more competence than you or I to decide, for example, which of competing candidates should have access to a kidney machine in the context of a scarcity of resources. The answer will be offered that the kidney machine goes to the patient medically most suited, but this is patently question begging, particularly when such factors as psychological stability and ability to comprehend and follow the necessary regime of food and behaviour are considered. Clearly, doctors must be the arbiters of those questions which are technical. Thereafter, the issue is an ethical one, even including the question of how far such technical information is to be deemed relevant to the conclusion to be reached. It may be that the solution which is least objectionable is a lottery, though many would object. A lottery was for instance used to allocate polio vaccine in England when it was first introduced and supplies were scarce. It is no answer to say that the real solution is the provision of enough machines for all, since this itself is part of a larger question concerning the allocation of resources among competing claims.

Victor Parsons and P. Lock show in their study published in the December 1980 issue of the *Journal of Medical Ethics* that the decisions which have to be made at present are agonisingly difficult for doctors. It seems quite unfair to place doctors in such a position. Their study consisted of a questionnaire sent to twenty-five renal dialysis units in the United Kingdom. Each unit was given the particulars of forty patients and told that ten would have to be rejected. Parsons and Lock write that many of the doctors "wrote long qualifying letters expressing their anxiety". "Only one physician", they report, "felt unable to reject any of the patients suggested on medical grounds." In the event, the results of the study were that "only 13 patients out of forty, i.e., one third, stood the chance of being accepted in all the units questioned; on the other hand no single patient in the series was rejected by all unit physicians. When we came to analyse the ten patients most frequently rejected, we found that at least six of them had been successfully treated by our own unit" (the cases were each based on real clinical practice).

A further ethical implication of the resort to advanced technology in medicine is the effect it may have on the way medicine and the doctor–patient relationship are conceived of by the doctor. The machine interposes itself between the doctor and the patient. It is relied upon. Any errors or misfortunes are its doing. Successes are the doctor's. The graveyard humour of "the operation was a success but the patient died" takes on a new significance when it is argued that the technique is perfectly sound but the patient did not respond to treatment. The engineer scientist model is reinforced at the expense of the model of the caring partner. Indeed, the machine may even become the end in itself, the *raison d'être* of the doctor, so that we may be persuaded to screen everyone for a susceptibility to a particular illness or abnormality without being in any way able to do anything with the information gained. In passing, it is interesting to wonder whether we are not seeing social history repeating itself here. Modern medicine, as we have seen, finds itself faced by and large with intractable conditions for which it can offer palliative measures at best. The days of conquest and cure on any large scale are gone. We are in a sense back in the state we were in before the major eradication of infectious diseases in the nineteenth and early twentieth centuries. Technology may be our modern witchcraft. We place the machine between us and the person complaining of being ill. The expert is trusted and relied upon. Sometimes the person gets well or improves, and we praise the wonders of technology. Sometimes he does not and we reassure ourselves that we did our best. I do not push the metaphor too far, but I offer it as worth consideration.

What remains then is for us to consider how to respond to the kind of ethical dilemmas I have alluded to. The answer, put in its simplest form, is that we, as lay people, must exercise some control. Those who develop and apply technology in medicine must be held accountable to all of us. I interject immediately that by control I do not mean prohibition or some heavy-handed bureaucratic machine. I mean that some mechanism must be created and established which is independent of any particular interest. Its role must be to lay down guidelines by reference to which the appropriate ethical decisions can be made. The crucial first task of this independent body would be to call for and disseminate information. By and large, the ethical problems we face are a consequence of technology being developed and introduced without any general awareness. What I contemplate is measured debate both before research is undertaken and before technology is introduced. This can only take place if information, on what is being done and what it may involve, is available to all. And in this context, as in many others, information is power, the first necessary step towards control.

The question then arises as to how a body such as the one I have suggested, on which an appropriately broad spectrum of opinion will be represented, will exercise control. No one wants to see government, or medicine, by committee. What I envisage is that after the first task, that of informing, is accomplished, issues of a general nature will be laid before this body of people and there debated. Comments would be invited from interested persons. Then guidelines would be produced which would serve as operating criteria according to which the research could be undertaken or the technology put into operation. It may be objected that this is a rather elaborate and slow process. But it is not beyond the wit of man to build a system which can operate successfully. Furthermore, time taken to debate the opening of the bottle is well spent if it means that the evil genie stays inside. The inquiry in 1978 into the siting of a nuclear power station conducted by Mr Justice Parker allowed the whole future of the use of nuclear energy in the United Kingdom to be debated and provides a model. That all did not approve of the final decisions does not invalidate the success of the enterprise. And of course such a large inquiry would be the exception rather than the rule, necessary when matters of the greatest significance for the future were involved.

Let me now turn to the dilemmas of modern medicine surrounding the end of life. I will concentrate on two issues – caring for the dying and the determination of death. It must be one of the most banal of statements to say that we must all die. But it seems sometimes as if we need to be reminded of the fact. *The Times* of 14 December 1976 heralded public discussion of death and dying as breaking "The last taboo". But the taboo is far from broken. It could be said that our interest is that of the voyeur and it coexists with that other part of our modern way of thinking, the denial of death, or at least the refusal to give it much thought, as being something that happens to others. The voyeur in us, for example, makes world-wide news of such commonplace tragedies as that of Karen Quinlan, just another girl who, through drugs or alcohol or both, ended up on a respirator in hospital. But that part of us which denies the inevitability of death prevents us from examining the facts, analysing what ought to be done, and suggesting remedies. We are content to say "poor thing" and wait for the next news item.

This sort of ambivalence is most obvious in the United States where there has been such an amazing outpouring of books, papers, newspaper articles and television programmes about death that it may be one of the liveliest growth industries in American letters. Yet, alongside this, the latest fad to preserve life, whether it be ginseng or jogging, sends this same middle-class voyeur off on another pursuit of Xanadu. Clinging to life reaches its high point in the lunatic fringe's conversion to cryogenics, whereby people are frozen after death to await some cure for that which killed them. Do not blame me for the logic. I am just repeating the argument. Jessica Mitford's biting commentary in *The American Way of Death* has not lost its validity. If anything has changed, it is merely that the death industry has become more respectable and intellectualised.

Perhaps the most important insight into the process of caring for the dying is that dying has become, to many, an illness. Call something an illness and you convert it into something which may respond to treatment, can even, perhaps, be cured. Add to this the doctor's claim that you cannot be sure that someone is dying – "he may recover, others have" – and you set the scene for a medical denial of death to complement the layman's. Death becomes like illness and disease, something to be defeated. The battle is not lost while there is something more which can be done. This is the point. We are in danger of seeing dying as something the doctor has to do something about, to try to prevent. We tend to expect this as an extension of our own anxieties and by medicalising dying the doctor is trapped by his own claim to expertise. Since a very large proportion of those who die do so now in hospital, this process of the medicalisation of death has inevitably gained momentum. Indeed, being in hospital the dying person confronts a medical attitude which will inevitably reflect the values of medicine which I have been describing. For, in general, it is the hospital doctor who *par excellence* considers himself the scientist problem-solver. There is a danger that dying comes to be seen as just another problem to be solved. Death is in a real sense a failure, not to be allowed without a fight. And, when you add into the equation the existence of the paraphernalia of the modern technology of life support, you supply the doctor with the tools with which to act out this communal denial of death.

It was Professor Henry Miller who railed against the sight of elderly patients existing in the twilight zone between life and death but not allowed to cross into the shadow because of the wonders of modern medicine. In the November 1967 *Proceedings* of the Royal Society of Medicine Professor Miller wrote that "there must be very few doctors who have not from time to time felt uneasiness, if not revulsion, at the spectacle of some stuporous ancient in hospital being maintained in a state of suspended animation by all the sophisticated paraphernalia of modern resuscitation".

There has more recently been some conscious effort to move away from this unsightly exercise and to change the attitude of doctors and lay people. The Hospice Movement has grown up, pioneered by Dame Cicely Saunders. Patients enter the hospice to await death. The regime is one of care which emphasises concern for the spiritual and psychological state of the patient but sets its face against the kind of technological warfare traditional hospitals may indulge in. Crucially, the staff concentrate on easing any pain the dying person may have, whether physical or mental. Years of research with mood–elevating drugs and with drugs to ease pain and control unpleasant symptoms have produced a body of pharmacotherapeutic knowledge which leads hospice staff to argue that no one now need die in pain or misery. This may be true in theory and the "Brompton cocktail", a mixture of strong pain-killing drugs under the influence of which the patient slid to his death, should be a thing of the past. The harsh fact, however, is that the vast majority of dying people do not find their way into hospices. Rather they die in general hospitals, often only after all efforts have been exhausted, where the careful management of pain and attention to spiritual needs hospice-style is unlikely to be encountered.

The principal ethical issue involved in the care of the dying concerns the duty the doctor owes his patient once the view is reached that the patient is dying. Note that I put the question in the form of the doctor's duty. This is because in my view the key concept in understanding the ethical basis of the doctor–patient relationship is duty, a duty owed by the doctor to the patient. Now I know some will say that I beg the question by assuming that the patient is dying, whereas the doctor may not be able to know this with such assurance. I readily concede that there must be a grey area in which the prognosis for the patient cannot be stated with precision. At the same time I would argue that if the doctor were making his determination in good faith, free of the pressure of others, relatives, nurses or colleagues, and liberated from the self-image of himself as the scientist problem-solver to whom death is failure, the view that a particular patient is dying can indeed be arrived at in very many cases. In the hope of avoiding confusion let me offer a further clarification. There are of course patients whose illness is fatal but who are at present enjoying a remission or are still able to live their lives albeit within narrowing constraints. I exclude these from those I refer to here as dying. I have in mind instead those whose illness has reached a terminal stage and for whom remission is either no longer possible or bought at great cost in terms of suffering or hardship.

Once a patient is seen to be dying, the duty the doctor owes him is, in my view, best stated as the duty to make what remains of his life comfortable. This is the principal ethical and legal duty. It carries with it the counterpart that the doctor has a duty to desist from measures which are designed to do other than comfort the patient. Continued chemotherapy, for example, or radiotherapy in the case of a dying patient, accompanied as they are by discomfort, are not only un-called for but a breach of the doctor's duty to his patient. The doctor does not desist from treating his patient. What changes is the nature of the treatment which is provided.

Seen in this light, a question which fascinates so many, that of when it is proper to turn off a respirator, can be shown to be one of the more simple questions to answer and it may be worth dealing with it here in passing. You must place the patient on the respirator into one of four categories. The first comprises those patients who are dead. The respirator is merely filling a corpse with air. Provided the determination of death is properly made, something I shall consider shortly, the respirator can be turned off. In the second category is the person who needs the respirator to breathe and is irreversibly in a state of coma. Once the patient's condition is incontrovertibly established, the doctor must, from time to time, disconnect the patient from the respirator so as to test the ability of the patient to breathe for himself. If the patient can breathe for himself, the question then becomes one of keeping him comfortable. Should he then develop some infection such as pneumonia the doctor is entitled to decide that given the hopelessness of the patient's condition he is not obliged to intervene to treat the infection but that his duty is rather to let the patient die. If, however, the patient does not breathe for himself or does so in a manner which would not be consistent with remaining alive, the doctor is entitled to consider whether returning the patient to the respirator is called for. If the patient's condition is so irreversibly hopeless, the doctor is entitled to desist from returning him to the respirator. The doctor is not obliged to continue with measures which are pointless and hopeless in that the patient's condition shows no possibility of recovery from the coma. The ethical question thus becomes not one of turning off the respirator but rather of turning it back on again. A third class of patients consists of those for whom the prognosis is still in doubt or who, for the time being, for whatever reason, need the respirator to aid breathing. In these circumstances, the doctor's duty is to persist with the respirator until the patient recovers or reaches the stage in which the prognosis is hopeless. If it is the latter the respirator is a burden and an intrusion upon the patient as in the previous case and the doctor having turned it off to ascertain the patient's condition is entitled to desist from turning it back on. The final class consists of those patients who are fully conscious and otherwise competent but who for reasons of some illness, for example polio, cannot breathe for themselves. There can be no question here of turning off the respirator as it cannot be classified as a hopeless and burdensome imposition on a patient who but for the respirator would die a peaceful death. From this brief outline it can be seen that the ethically relevant decision is not whether to turn off the respirator. Rather, it is the decision whether to turn it back on again in the light of the prognosis arrived at concerning the particular patient.

The ethical duty of the doctor, therefore, in general terms, moves from the duty to maintain and preserve life to the duty to make the patient comfortable and avoid all intervention of a pointless and hopeless nature. This movement coincides with that of the patient from being categorised as ill and therefore capable of recovery, or at least not dying, to being categorised as dying. However, a powerful combination of factors all conspire to produce a situation in which the dying are not easily allowed to die. They include the training of doctors as problem-solvers, our cultural rejection or denial of death, pressure from relatives or, rarely, patients themselves, the existence of the technology to maintain a semblance of life and the enthusiasm, particularly of young doctors, to regard dying as a challenge to be overcome. "Rage, rage against the coming of the night" was how Dylan Thomas captured our inability to come to terms with death. The unseemly intervention of doctors, flown in from all over the world, in the dying agony of such figures as General Franco, President Tito and the Shah of Iran, and the morbid attention given to this by the press, radio and television, serve to reinforce this attitude.

It is no wonder that there have appeared movements concerned with "Death with Dignity" or "The Right to Die". This latter label is, of course, rather silly. Those supporting it do not really call for a right to die. We all die, right or no. What they really mean is the right to be allowed to die without further medical intervention. They call for the ultimate right to self-determination and control, the right to have your own death. It is no wonder either that there is renewed interest in voluntary euthanasia and in suicide, even to the point of a proposal by the organisation in the United Kingdom called Exit to publish a pamphlet for members containing instructions on effective self-destruction. The fear of languishing in the twilight state between life and death, as a medical preparation, a tribute to medical technology, is an important factor in bringing this about. Remove the fear, reassert the true nature of the doctor's duty and the need would disappear.

Of course, it is only right to notice that doctors often find themselves in an unenviable situation. Their view of their duty to the patient may be challenged by relatives who demand all efforts to be continued, hopeless though they may be. The doctor is damned if he continues and thereby breaches his duty. But he is damned if he does not, since the relatives may apply pressure, complain or even threaten him with a lawsuit for neglecting his patient. The problem is that it is hard to find any authoritative statement of society's decision as to the doctor's duty, whether in the form of law or otherwise. This lack of any clear guide allows the dilemmas I have identified to persist. I have no doubt that what I have said represents both the ethical and legal duty of the doctor. But clearly there is a need to state this view in some authoritative form. I would not have thought that this was a matter for the heavy hand of legislation, or even for a ruling in a case brought before the courts, although both solutions have been tried in the United States. What seems appropriate for the United Kingdom is the preparation, after due and general deliberation, of an appropriate code of practice. Doctors' jealous defence of what they mistakenly regard as their sphere of exclusive competence and the traditionally British attitude of muddling through have combined so far to prevent this from happening. But, if the price to be paid is unhappiness and misery and if the doctor has so much to gain from the help such a code would offer, it would be better if something were done and done soon.

I turn now to the definition and determination of death. It is a commonplace now that the modern medical technology of intensive care and life support has rendered the old ways of recognising death unreliable. It used to be said that death was the absence of vital functions. The vital functions which were thought to be particularly relevant were breathing, heartbeat and the capacity for consciousness. Now we all know that breathing and heartbeat can be maintained by machinery, so that this way of determining death may not be helpful in the case of patients who find themselves in intensive care units. It may not be the patient who is breathing. The patient may be in a coma and unable ever to breathe again. It may be the machine which is breathing for the patient. The machine may be ventilating a corpse. The machine may, in a word, mimic life. The question is how to analyse this intellectually, and how to discover it in fact.

Clearly, it is important to know when and whether someone is dead. Not only does he cease to be a person but our attitude to him changes completely. He is a corpse not a person. A doctor owes a corpse no duties, save perhaps decent respect. A corpse has no claims on anyone, nor any obligations. A living person is owed duties and can have obligations. The law of homicide calls for a dead body. The law of succession comes into operation only on death. We only bury people when they are dead. And, of limited importance, but crucial in focusing attention on the issue of death, we may not remove the organs of someone for the purposes of transplantation until that person is dead. Kidneys and other organs must however be removed fairly soon after death (within about an hour) if they are to be of use when transplanted. And there was some sense of unease, especially in the early days particularly of heart transplants, that maybe some medical sleight-of-hand was being practised. The need to determine the moment of death, hitherto not regarded as particularly crucial since time was no longer of the essence, became of the greatest significance.

There are in fact two problems involved in any analysis of the meaning of death. The first concerns the definition of death; the second, the determination that the state as defined is present. Let us consider the definition first. It cannot be stated too emphatically that the definition of death is not a scientific, technical matter. The definition of death is concerned with the point at which someone ceases to be a person. A person is someone whom the law protects, to whom duties are owed both legal and ethical, and who may make claims on others. What we are concerned with is the identification of that which is crucial to being a person. This is clearly a philosophical and spiritual issue. Scientific information is relevant in helping us to analyse the concept of personality. But it cannot, of itself, tell us what person-ality consists of. This calls for a judgement. The definition of death calls, therefore, for a normative judgement. It calls for the selection of a point beyond which we are prepared to say someone is no longer a person.

To speak of the selection of a point is to understand that a number of options might exist in a process that begins with birth. We could say that someone is no longer a person, is dead, only when he has completely and totally decomposed. We could say someone is dead when he is unconscious, in a coma from which he will never recover, even though he is still breathing. If consciousness were the key, we could say that someone who was so severely mentally retarded as to display no evidence of conscious awareness, or someone in an advanced state of senility, is dead. In mediaeval times, it may be recalled, entering the church was described as civil death. The person no longer existed according to the civil law.

Of the various choices available, the point at which death is deemed to occur has always been that point at which the vital functions of breathing, heartbeat and the capacity for consciousness have ceased for ever. This may have been because the heart was once regarded as the seat of the emotions and it was these which were identified as being the crucial feature of being a person. The heart is no longer thought of as being the seat of the emotions, except perhaps by the manufacturers of Valentine cards. The brain has supplanted it as that part of us in which are thought to reside the mind, the emotions, the spiritual sense of self. This might lead us to abandon heartbeat and breathing as the relevant criteria of personality, and thus of life and death, in favour of consciousness. But the difficulty with this is that consciousness can be lost for ever, but a person in such a condition may continue to breathe. This is because breathing and heartbeat do not depend for their continued functioning on that part of the brain responsible for conscious thought, the higher brain. Rather, it is the brain-stem, that part at the base and back of the brain, which is responsible for their continued functioning. So, if we were to regard permanent loss of consciousness as death, it would mean that someone would be dead who was breathing of his own accord. Clearly, this is unacceptable and the importance of the old notion of absence of vital functions reasserts itself. This has led some to argue for a definition of death which calls for the destruction of the higher brain *and* the brain-stem, so-called total brain death. The notion of personality shifted, therefore, from the heart to the total brain. But there is something wrong with this analysis. The brain-stem is not only responsible for maintaining breathing and heartbeat. It is also responsible for the continued capacity to function of the higher brain in which consciousness resides. The brain-stem is akin to the body's switchboard. All signals go through it. If it is destroyed, nothing can function. There can be no breathing, no heartbeat, no thought. Thus it was concluded that what is crucial to personality is the brain-stem since it is the brain-stem which maintains all vital functions. Death on this basis, therefore, is the total and irreversible loss of all brain-stem function. Furthermore, this definition does no violence to the traditional notion of death, the absence of vital functions. All it does is to allow the absence of these functions to be identified when otherwise they may be thought still to exist because a patient is being maintained on a respirator which is breathing for him and making his heart beat.

Some are uneasy about this definition. They are reluctant to make the step from total brain death to brain-stem death. They persist in the view that the upper brain must be shown to be completely devoid of all electrical activity before someone can be regarded as dead. This view, in the opinion of many, is unwarranted. It fails to take account of the fact that the upper brain's ability to function is dependent on the brain-stem. And it argues for a new definition of death.

Let me explain this second criticism. What concerns those who argue for total brain death is that even where the destruction of the brain-stem can be established it is still possible on occasions to monitor electrical activity in the higher brain. Only when this activity has ceased for ever, they argue, should a person be regarded as dead. The objection to this line of argument is that what is being monitored is spontaneous electrical activity which may well persist after the death of a person. After all, the hair and finger nails of a corpse will continue to grow after death. We do not wait until they have stopped growing before declaring death. Nor do we need to wait for every trace of electrical discharge in the higher brain to have disappeared. To do so would confuse the death of a person with the subsequent death of parts of his body, in this case his higher brain, which we have already noticed cannot have the capacity to be conscious once the brain-stem is destroyed. It would mean that a new definition of death, quite distinct from the notion of absence of vital functions, was being advocated.

Clearly, if brain-stem death represented in fact a *new* definition of death, it would not be for doctors or medical scientists to decide upon and adopt it. Given that death represents a fundamental judgement about the nature of life and personality, it would be for all of us to debate and discuss before any new definition were accepted. But, for the reasons I have given, I do not regard brain-stem death as a new definition of death. Rather, I see it as a new method of identifying that which we have always regarded as death, made necessary by the fact that machines can now mimic life. It is the relatively small number of adherents of total brain death who are in fact advocating a new definition of death, even though they purport to be defending the traditional definition. Their view has been rejected, at least in the United Kingdom. In 1976 the Royal Colleges of Medicine endorsed the concept of brain-stem death, reaffirming that it was no more than another way of expressing the traditional notion of death as being the absence of vital functions.

Once the definitional choice is made, the process of determining its existence is a relatively simple technical exercise. In their report on brain-stem death, published in the *British Medical Journal* of 13 November 1976, the Royal Colleges laid down a code of practice to be followed in determining the presence of brain-stem death. The procedures are carefully designed to provide for the elimination of conditions which could be mistaken for brain-stem death, especially intoxication of the patient from drugs or alcohol or the presence of hypothermia as the cause of the patient's coma. One procedure which is not called for in the British code of practice is the need to take a tracing of the electrical activity of the higher brain by means of an electroencephalograph. Some criticise this as a weakness in the code, but the criticism is ill conceived. As we have seen, death is to be determined by reference to the destruction of the brain-stem not the higher brain. And electroencephalography is quite simply irrelevant to this exercise, since the presence of

electrical activity in the higher brain cannot be associated
with consciousness once the brain-stem is destroyed.

Although I have described the test for determining brain-
stem death as a relatively simple exercise, it is, of course,
vital that it be carried out competently by appropriately
qualified doctors. Once it has been carried out and death
confirmed, all the apparatus of life support can, of course,
be removed. This may unnerve some, since the heart of the
patient is still beating. Once it is realised that it is the
machinery and not the person which is making the heart
beat, the problem is resolved. And, in any event, when
brain-stem death has occurred, the heart will cease beating
within a matter of a few days even if the life-support
machinery is not turned off.

Finally, it is right to say that satisfactory as the British
code is, both in concept and detail, there is one area in which
it ought to be amended. At present, there are no provisions
which specify the time after the onset of the patient's coma
at which the test should be carried out nor the appropriate
intervals of time which should elapse before a further
confirmatory test is carried out. There are only recommendations. Indeed, there is no requirement that the original
diagnosis be confirmed, although the code notes that it is
customary to do so and recommends it be done. Clearly, in
some cases, there is no need to wait to carry out the test.
When a patient is admitted to intensive care who has been
all but decapitated in a road accident, there can be little
question about the confirmation of brain-stem death. On
the other hand there may be circumstances in which the
patient's coma may be caused by a variety of factors,
including drug intoxication. In such a case it may be decided
that a more obvious factor – for example severe head injury
– is the cause of the coma, and consequently the possible
relevance of the drugs could be overlooked. The difficulty is
that drug intoxication can, for a short period, produce an
impression of brain-stem death. Too hasty a decision to
diagnose brain-stem death may be made. The possibility

that the patient's condition could be treated, once the effect of the drug intoxication had disappeared, would be overlooked.

There is in my view a need to revise the code to respond to this possibility, unusual though it may be. Specific provisions must be incorporated into the code setting out the time which should elapse before carrying out the test, so as to establish without doubt the cause of the coma. A confirmatory test is not of course necessary strictly speaking if the first test is properly carried out. Nonetheless a provision requiring a confirmatory test and setting out the time interval which should elapse before it is carried out could be incorporated if it were thought appropriate. Only in this way will the residual doubts of a public not yet fully accustomed to the notion of brain-stem death be allayed and the possibility of occasional misdiagnosis be avoided.

Conclusion

In these chapters I have examined some of the dilemmas of modern medicine as I see them. I have sought to unmask medicine. I do not suggest there is anything sinister underneath. There is something of value for all of us once we dispel some of the myths and fancies. I have suggested that there must be a new relationship between doctor and patient. I have suggested that we must take responsibility for our lives. I have suggested that we must challenge the power which doctors exert over our lives. I have suggested that doctors must be made accountable to us. I have suggested ways of redressing the balance of power. I have suggested ways in which a new partnership based on mutual respect may be forged. I have sought to start the debate. Now you must take over.

Bibliography

PRINCIPAL SOURCES

Doyal, Lesley, with Pennell, Imogen, *The Political Economy of Health*, Pluto Press, 1979.

Draper, Peter, *et al.*, *The NHS in the next 30 years: A new perspective on the health of the British*, Unit for the Study of Health Policy, Department of Community Medicine, Guy's Hospital Medical School, 1978.

Illich, Ivan, *Limits to Medicine*, Penguin, 1977.

Inequalities in Health: Report of a Research Working Group, D.H.S.S., 1980.

McKeown, Thomas, *The Role of Medicine*, Basil Blackwell, 1979.

Miller, Henry, *Medicine and Society*, Oxford University Press, 1973.

Muir Gray, J. A., *Man Against Disease: Preventive Medicine*, Oxford University Press, 1979.

Report of the Royal Commission on the National Health Service, Cmnd. 7615, H.M.S.O., 1979.

Wilson, Michael, *Health is for People*, Darton, Longman & Todd, 1975.

The extensive notes and bibliographies in these works are an invaluable source of further material.

SUPPLEMENTARY READING

Black, Douglas, *"Cui bono?"*, *British Medical Journal*, 29 October, 1977, pp. 1109–14.

Black, D., "Client–oriented medicine", in *Research and Medical Practice: their interaction*, Ciba Foundation, 1976.

Brenner, M. H., *Estimating The Social Costs of National Economic Policy*, U.S. Government Printing Office, 1976.

Campbell, E. J. M., *et al.*, "The concept of disease", *British Medical Journal*, 29 September 1979, Vol. 2, pp. 757–62.

Cobbs v. *Grant* (1972) 104 Cal. Rptr. 505, 502 P. 2d 1.

Cochrane, A. L., *Effectiveness and Efficiency: Random Reflections on Health Services*, London, Nuffield Provincial Hospitals Trust/Oxford University Press, 1972.

Davis, Alan, *Relationships Between Doctors and Patients*, Saxon House reprint, Teakfield, 1978.

Dubos, René, *The Mirage of Health*, Allen & Unwin, 1970.

Duff, Raymond, "Guidelines for Deciding Care of Critically Ill or Dying Patients", *Pediatrics*, Vol. 64, No. 1, July 1979.

Duff, Raymond, and Campbell, A. G. M., "Moral and Ethical Dilemmas in the Special-care Nursery", *New England Journal of Medicine*, Vol. 289, No. 17, 25 October 1973, pp. 890–4.

Duncan, A. S., *et al.* (eds), *Dictionary of Medical Ethics*, Darton, Longman & Todd, 1981.

"Fit for the Future", Report of the Committee on the Child Health Services, (Cmnd. 6684), London, H.M.S.O., 1976.

Foucault, Michel, *The Birth of the Clinic*, Tavistock Publications, 1973.

Freund, P. (ed.), *Experimentation with Human Subjects*, George Braziller, New York, 1969.

Gaylin, Willard, "In matters mental or emotional What's Normal?", *New York Times Magazine*, 1 April 1973, pp. 14, 54, 56–57.

Glover, Jonathan, *Causing Deaths and Saving Lives*, Penguin, 1977.

The Handbook of Medical Ethics, British Medical Association, 1980.

Jones, Alun, and Bodmer, Walter F., *Our Future Inheritance: Choice or Chance?*, Oxford University Press, 1974.

Katz, Jay, *Experimentation with Human Beings*, Russell Sage Foundation, New York, 1972.

Lalonde, M., *A New Perspective on the Health of Canadians*, Government of Canada, 1974.

Liacos, Paul, "Dilemmas of Dying", *Medicolegal News*, Fall 1979, pp. 4–7 and 29.

Lorber, J., "Selective treatment of myelomeningocele", *Pediatrics*, Vol. 53, No. 3, March 1974, pp. 307–8.

MacIntyre, Alasdair, "Why is the Search for the Foundations of Ethics so Frustrating?", *The Hastings Center Report*, August 1979.

Parsons, T., "Health and Society", *British Medical Journal*, 1975, 53, p. 257.

People v. *Privitera*, 591 P. 2d, 919 (Cal. 1979).

Pickering, Sir George, *Quest for Excellence in Medical Education*, published for Nuffield Provincial Hospitals Trust by Oxford University Press, 1978.

Powledge, Tabitha, and Fletcher, John, "Guidelines for the Ethical, Social and Legal Issues in Prenatal Diagnosis", *New England Journal of Medicine*, Vol. 300, pp. 168–72, 25 January 1979.

Powles, J., "On the Limitations of Modern Medicine", *Science, Medicine and Man*, 1. 1:1.

In re Quinlan, 70 N.J. 10 (1976).

Ramsey, Paul, *The Patient as Person*, Yale University Press, 1970.

Reiser, Stanley Joel, Dyck, Arthur J., Curran, William J. (eds), *Ethics in Medicine: Historical Perspectives and Contemporary Concerns*, M.I.T. Press, Cambridge, Massachusetts, 1977.

Relman, Arnold, "The Saikewicz Decision: Judges as Physicians", *New England Journal of Medicine*, Vol. 298, No. 9, March 1978, pp. 508–9.

Robertson, John, "Involuntary Euthanasia of Defective Newborns: A Legal Analysis", *Stanford Law Review*, Vol. 27, January 1975, pp. 213–9.

Robinson, David, *The Process of Becoming Ill*, Routledge & Kegan Paul, 1971.

Rollin, Bernard E., "On the Nature of Illness", *Man and Medicine*, Vol. 4, No. 3, 1979, pp. 157–72.

Sontag, Susan, *Illness as Metaphor*, Penguin, 1977.

Specialized Futures: Essays in Honour of Sir George Goodber, GCB, published for The Nuffield Provincial Hospitals Trust by the Oxford University Press, 1975.

Superintendent of Belchertown State School v. *Saikewicz*, 370 N.E. 2d 417 (Mass. 1977).

Swinyard, Chester A. (ed.), *Decision Making and The Defective Newborn*, Charles C. Thomas, Springfield, Illinois, 1978.

Szasz, Thomas, *The Theology of Medicine*, Oxford University Press, 1979.

Szasz, Thomas, *The Myth of Mental Illness*, Paladin, 1962.

Veatch, Robert, *Death, Dying, and the Biological Revolution*, Yale University Press, 1976.

Whitehouse v. *Jordan*, (1980), 1A11 E.R., 650.

Wildavsky, A., in Knowles, J. H. (ed.), *Doing Better and Feeling Worse*, American Acad. of Arts and Sciences, 1977.

Wolstenholme, G. E. W., and O'Connor, M. (eds), *Ethics in Medical Progress, with special reference to transplantation*, CIBA Foundation Symposium, J. A. Churchill, 1966.

Working party of the Newcastle Regional Hospital Board, "Ethics of Selective Treatment of Spina Bifida", *The Lancet*, 11 January 1975, pp. 85–8.

Each of these works has notes and bibliographies for further reading.

GENERAL READING

These are in addition to the books, papers, notes and bibliographies already referred to. They are organised under headings which are intended to serve merely as guides.

Ethics

(i) General

Hampshire, Stuart (ed.), *Public and Private Morality*, Cambridge University Press, 1978.

Putnam, Hilary, *Meaning and the Moral Sciences*, Routledge & Kegan Paul, 1978.

Singer, Peter, *Practical Ethics,* Cambridge University Press, 1979.
Warnock, Mary, *Ethics Since 1900,* Oxford University Press, 1978.

(ii) Medical Ethics

Alting von Geusau, F. A. M., de Locht, P., Dumas, A., and Hellegers, A., *Biology, Ethics and Society: Questions and Issues,* Prospective International, Brussels, 1979.

Beauchamp, Tom L., and Childress, James F., *Principles of Biomedical Ethics,* Oxford University Press, New York, 1979.

Beecher, Henry, "Ethics and Clinical Research", *New England Journal of Medicine,* Vol. 274, pp. 1354–60, 1966.

Campbell, A. V., *Moral Dilemmas in Medicine,* Churchill Livingstone, 1972.

Capron, Alexander, "Medical Research in Prisons", *The Hastings Center Report,* No. 6, 1973, pp. 4–7.

CIBA Foundation Symposium 16, *Medical Care of Prisoners and Detainees,* Elsevier, *Excerpta Medica,* North-Holland, 1973.

A Conversation With Dr. Leon Kass: The Ethical Dimensions of in Vitro Fertilization, American Enterprise Institute for Public Policy Research, Washington, D.C., 1979.

Cooper, Theodore, "The Challenge to the Medical Profession", *New England Journal of Medicine,* Vol. 300, No. 21, pp. 1185–8, 24 May 1979.

Curran, William, and Beecher, Henry, "Experimentation in Children", *Journal of the American Medical Association,* Vol. 10, No. 1, 6 October 1969, pp. 77–83.

Danielli, James F., "Industry, Society, and Genetic Engineering",The Hastings Center, Readings of the Institute of Society, Ethics and the Life Sciences, 1972.

Davis, John W., Hoffmaster, Barry, and Shorten, Sarah, *Contemporary Issues in Biomedical Ethics,* The Humana Press, New Jersey, 1978.

Dickens, Bernard M., "Guidelines on The Use of Human Subjects", Office of Research Administration, University of Toronto, 1979.

Green, Richard, and Money, John (eds), *Transsexualism and Sex Reassignment,* Johns Hopkins Press, Baltimore, Maryland, 1969.

Gustafson, James, in Williams, Preston N. (ed.), "Genetic Engineering and the Normative View of the Human", *Ethical Issues in Biology and Medicine,* Schenkman, 1973.

Hodges, Lucy, "Protest to minister on use of drugs to calm children in home", *The Times,* 28 May 1980.

Lappé, Marc, "Moral Obligations and the Fallacies of 'Genetic Control' ", *Theological Studies,* Vol. 33, No. 3, September 1972, pp. 411–27.

Lorber, J., "Results of Treatment of Myelomeningocele", *Developmental Medicine and Child Neurology,* 1971, 13, pp. 279–303.

Neville, Robert, "Ethical and Philosophical Issues of Behavior Control", presented at the 139th Annual Meeting of The American Association for The Advancement of Science, 27 December 1972.

Pub. Law 93–348. *Title II – Protection of Human Subjects of Biomedical and Behavioral Research*, 12 July 1974, 93rd Congress, H.R. 7724, 88 Stat. 348.

Ramsey, Paul, *Ethics at the Edges of Life*, Yale University Press, 1978.

Ramsey, Paul, *The Ethics of Fetal Research*, Yale University Press, 1975.

Ramsey, Paul, "Genetic Therapy: A Theologian's Response", in Hamilton, Michael P. (ed.), *The New Genetics and the Future of Man*, chapter 8, Eerdmans, 1972.

Ryan, Michael, "Ethics and the patient with cancer", *British Medical Journal*, 25 August 1979, pp. 480–1.

Stoller, Robert J., *Sex and Gender*, Science House, New York, 1968.

Thomas, Lewis, "The Technology of Medicine", *New England Journal of Medicine*, 285 (1971), 1366.

Veatch, Robert, and Sollitto, Sharmon, "Human Experimentation – The Ethical Questions Persist", *The Hastings Center Report*, Vol. 3, No. 3, June 1973, pp. 1–3.

Visscher, Maurice B. (ed.), *Humanistic Perspectives in Medical Ethics*, Prometheus Books, Buffalo, 1972.

(iii) Costs, Benefits and Risks

Bailey, Martin J., *Reducing Risks to Life: Measurement of the Benefits*, American Enterprise Institute for Public Policy Research, Washington, D.C., 1980.

Calabresi, Guido, "The Decision for Accidents: An Approach to Non-Fault Allocation of Costs", *Harvard Law Review*, 1965.

Card, W. I., and Mooney, G. H., "What is the monetary value of a human life?", *British Medical Journal*, 24–31 December 1977, Vol. 2, pp. 1627–9.

Comment, "Considerations in the Regulation of Biological Research", *University of Pennsylvania Law Review*, Vol. 126, 1420–46, 1978.

Ferguson, James R., "Scientific Inquiry and The First Amendment", *Cornell Law Review*, Vol. 64, 639–65, 1979.

Golding, A. M. B., and Tosey, D., "The Cost of High Technology Medicine", *The Lancet*, 26 July 1980, pp. 195–7.

"Heart Transplants back in favour, surgeon says", *The Times*, 12 September 1980.

Kay, H. E. M., *et al.*, "Cost of Bone-Marrow Transplants in Acute Myeloid Leukaemia", *The Lancet*, 17 May 1980, pp. 1067–9.

Knox, Richard A., "Heart Transplants: To Pay or Not to Pay", *Science*, Vol. 209, 1 August 1980, pp. 570–5.

Knox, Richard A., "Mass. General: No Heart Transplants Here", *Science*, Vol. 209, 1 August 1980, p. 574.

Miller, J., and Yandle, B. (eds), *Benefit–Cost Analyses of Social Regulation*, American Enterprise Institute for Public Policy Research, Washington, D.C., 1979.

Morley, David, *The Sensitive Scientist*, S.C.M. Press, 1978.

Powles, R. L., *et al.*, "The Place of Bone-Marrow Transplantation in Acute Lyelogeneus Leukaemia", *The Lancet*, 17 May 1980, pp. 1047–50.

Ross, Walter S., *The Life/Death Ratio*, Readers Digest Press, New York, 1977.

Sauer, Loie, "Before Proof of Cancer, 'High Risk' Women Opt for Breast Surgery", *New York Times*, 23 September 1980.

Swets, John, *et al.*, "Assessment of Diagnostic Technologies", *Science*, 24 August 1979, Vol. 205, No. 4407, pp. 753–9.

Woodruff, Professor Sir Michael, *Edwin Stevens Lectures for the Laity: "The One and the Many"*, Royal Society of Medicine, 1970.

Wright, Pearce, "New formula costs cancer deaths", *The Times*, 20 March 1980.

Philosophy of Medicine

Blakemore, Colin, *Mechanics of the Mind*, Cambridge University Press, 1976.

Churchland, Patricia Smith, "A Perspective on Mind–Brain Research", *The Journal of Philosophy*, Vol. LXXVII, No. 4, April 1980, pp. 185–207.

Comment, "When is a disease not a disease?", *Science News*, Vol. 118.

Engelhardt, H. Tristam, and Spicker, Stuart F., *Evaluation and Explanation in the Biomedical Sciences*, D. Reidel Publishing Company, Dordrecht, Holland, 1975.

Fletcher, Joseph, "Indicators of Humanhood: A Tentative Profile of Man", *The Hastings Center Report*, Vol. 2, No. 5, November 1972, pp. 1–4.

Huxley, Andrew, "Evidence, Clues, and Motive in Science", B.A. Presidential Address, 139th Annual Meeting of the British Association for the Advancement of Science, 31 August–7 September 1977.

Kraupl Taylor, F., *The Concepts of Illness, Disease and Morbus*, Cambridge University Press, 1979.

Nagel, Thomas, *Mortal Questions*, Cambridge University Press, 1979.

Sennett, Richard, "Books: The Desire to Know", *The New Yorker*, 16 July 1979, pp. 101–6.

Young, J. Z., *Programs of The Brain*, Oxford University Press, 1978.

Medical Sociology

Baechler, Jean, *Suicides*, Basil Blackwell, Oxford, 1979.

Cousins, Norman, *Anatomy of An Illness*, W. W. Norton & Co., New York, 1979.

Gerson, E. M., "Social Science and Medicine", *British Medical Journal*, 1976, 10, p. 219.

Kitwood, Tom, *Disclosures to a Stranger*, Routledge & Kegan Paul, 1980.

Loraine, John A., *Global Signposts to the 21st Century*, Peter Owen, 1979.

Renvoize, Jean, *Children in Danger*, Routledge & Kegan Paul, 1974.

Ryan, Michael, *The Organization of Soviet Medical Care*, Basil Blackwell, Oxford, and Martin Robertson, London, 1978.

Schofield, Michael, *The Strange Case of Pot*, Penguin, 1971.

Shennan, Victoria, *Mental Handicap Nursing and Care*, Souvenir Press, 1980.

Tiger, Lionel, *Optimism: The Biology of Hope*, Secker & Warburg, 1979.

Titmuss, Richard M., *The Gift Relationship*, Pantheon Books, New York, 1971.

Tuckett, D., *An Introduction to Medical Sociology*, London, Tavistock Publications, 1976.

Medical Law and Legal Theory

Bevan, H. K., *The Law Relating to Children*, Butterworth, 1973.

Cook, R. J., and Dickens, B. M., *Abortion Laws in Commonwealth Countries*, World Health Organisation, Geneva, 1979.

Curran, William J., and Shapiro, E. Donald, *Law, Medicine, and Forensic Science*, Little, Brown and Co., Boston, 1970.

Dickens, Bernard M., *Medico-Legal Aspects of Family Law*, Butterworth, Toronto, 1979.

King, Joseph, *The Law of Medical Malpractice in a Nutshell*, West Publishing Co., 1977.

Law and the Doctor, The Medical Defence Union, 1975.

The Law Reform Commission, *Human Tissue Transplants*, Report No. 7, Australian Government Publishing Service, Canberra, 1977.

Lloyd, D., *The Idea of Law*, Penguin, 1964.

Lloyd, D., *Introduction to Jurisprudence*, Stevens, 1979.

McClean, J. D., *The Legal Context of Social Work*, Butterworth, 1975.

Meyers, David W., *The Human Body and The Law*, Aldine, Chicago, 1970.

National Assistance Act, 1948, section 47.

Norman, Alison J., *Rights & Risk*, National Corporation for the Care of Old People, London, 1980.

Ontario Interministerial Committee on Medical Consent, *Options on Medical Consent*, 1979.

Paxman, John (ed.), *Law and Planned Parenthood*, International Planned Parenthood Federation, 1980.

Report of The International Conference on the Legal and Ethical Aspects of Health Care for Children, Ontario, 25–7 October 1979.

"The Right to Refuse Psychoactive Drugs", *The Hastings Center Report*, No. 6, 1973, Institute of Society, Ethics, and the Life Sciences, pp. 8–11.

Speller, S. R., *Law of Doctor and Patient*, H. K. Lewis, 1973.

Stetler, C. Joseph, and Moritz, Alan R., *Doctor and Patient and the Law*, C. V. Mosby Company, Saint Louis, Missouri, 1962.

Taylor, N. L., *Doctors and The Law*, Oyez Publishing, 1976.

Williams, Glanville, *The Sanctity of Life and the Criminal Law*, Faber & Faber, 1958.

Wood, Clive (ed.), *The Influence of Litigation on Medical Practice*, Academic Press, 1977.

Politics of Health

Ashley, Jack, and Hannam, John, letter to editor, *The Times*, 1 June 1980.

"Assurance on invalidity benefit subject to available resources", *The Times*, 22 May 1980.

Battye, G. C., "Unemployment and Health", *The Lancet*, 7 April 1979, p. 780.

Brenner, M. Harvey, "Mortality and the National Economy", *The Lancet*, 15 September 1979, pp. 568–73.

Brenner, M. Harvey, "Unemployment, Economic Growth, and Mortality", *The Lancet*, 24 March 1979, p. 672.

Brewster Kingman, *Edwin Stevens Lectures for the Laity: "Health At Any Price?"* Royal Society of Medicine, 1980.

Brown, E. Richard, *Rockefeller Medicine Men*, University of California Press, Berkeley, 1979.

Bunn, Rex, "Unemployment, Morbidity, and Mortality", *The Lancet*, 28 April 1979, pp. 923–4.

"Child Benefit should be top priority", *The Times*, 29 July 1980.

Draper, Peter, "How Can We Make Progress in Health?", presented at the Annual Meeting of the British Association for the Advancement of Science, 1–5 September 1980.

Draper, P., *et al.*, "Micro-Processors, Macro Economic Policy, and Public Health", *The Lancet*, Vol. i, p. 373, 1979.

Erikkson, Jan, *et al.*, 'Unemployment and Health", *The Lancet*, 2 June 1979, p. 1189.

Ferriman, Annabel, "Family man will be more than £3 a week worse off in sickness pay under government proposal", *The Times*, 3 April 1980.

Ferriman, Annabel, "Leukaemia victims die for lack of facilities", *The Times*, 17 June 1980.

Ferriman, Annabel, "Minister rebuked on health report", *The Times*, 30 August 1980.

176 *The Unmasking of Medicine*

Health: Sector Policy Paper, World Bank, 1980.

Healy, Pat, "Grant cuts affect poor families", *The Times*, 18 June 1980.

Healy, Pat, "Social Security: the Government goes back to basics", *The Times*, 21 May 1980.

Hebert, Hugh, "Call for better child care likely to go unheeded", *Guardian*, 29 August 1980.

Hebert, Hugh, "Care worn", *Guardian*, 29 August 1980.

Homeless and Healthless, City and Hackney Community Health Council, 1978.

Jobling, R. G., "Unemployment and Health", *The Lancet*, 2 June 1979, p. 1189.

Marchasin, Sidney, "Laetrile: Out of the Lab, Into the Legislature", *Los Angeles Times*, 30 March 1980.

Meyer, Jack A., *Health Care Cost Increase*, American Enterprise Institute for Public Policy Research, Washington, D.C., 1979.

"More young people to pay for dental treatment", *The Times*, 11 June 1980.

Morris, J. N., "Equalities and Inequalities in Health", *British Medical Journal*, Vol. 281, 11 October 1980, p. 1003.

Morris, J. N., "Social Inequalities Diminished", *Health Visitor*, Vol. 53, September 1980, reprinted from *The Lancet*, 1979, i, 87–90.

Osman, Arthur, "Best hospital care for 'women least in need' ", *The Times*, 15 April 1980.

"Patients First", Department of Health and Social Security, Welsh Office, Consultative paper on the structure and management of The National Health Service in England and Wales, H.M.S.O., London, 1979.

Privitera, James, "Out of Jail, Back in the Fight", *Los Angeles Times*, 30 March 1980.

Roper, John, "Can private medicine help the Health Service out of its present difficulties?", *The Times*, 10 January 1980.

Scott-Samuel, Alex, "Unemployment and Health", *The Lancet*, 3 March 1979, p. 498.

"Does Unemployment Kill?", *The Lancet*, 31 March 1979, pp. 708–9.

Unit for the Study of Health Policy, "Effective Prevention: A Comparative Analysis", a short description of a three-year research project unit for the study of health policy, Department of Community Medicine, Guy's Hospital Medical School, 1980.

Wechster, Henry, Gurin, Joel, and Cahill, George F., *The Horizons of Health*, Harvard University Press, Cambridge, Massachusetts, 1977.

Wildavsky, Aaron, "Wealthier is Healthier", *Regulation, AEI Journal on Government and Society*, January/February 1980, pp. 10–12 and 55.

Wilson, Michael, *Health is for People*, Darton, Longman & Todd, 1975.

Young, Robin, "Low Paid: Hidden snags leave some worse off", *The Times*, 27 March 1980.

Preventive Medicine/Promotion of Health

"Appeal for funds to study back pain", *The Times*, 15 September 1980.

Ball, Keith, letter to editor on prevention of coronary heart disease, *The Lancet*, 1 December 1979, p. 1182.

Burkitt, Denis, letter to the editor, *The Times*, 11 September 1980.

Chemical Industries Association, *Cancer in Modern Mortality*, White Crescent Press, 1978.

Department of Trade, *Personal Factors in Domestic Accidents, Prevention Through Product and Environmental Design*, Consumer Safety Unit, 1980.

Ferriman, Annabel, "Compulsory wearing of seat belts 'inevitable' ", *The Times*, 12 June 1980.

Ferriman, Annabel, "Doctors condemn low tax rises on tobacco and alcohol and propose a ban on public smoking", *The Times*, 9 July 1980.

Ferriman, Annabel, "Smokers resist change of habit", *The Times*, 10 January 1980.

Gibbs, Frances, "Screening for early diagnosis", *The Times*, 21 February 1980.

Havighurst, C., and Hackbarth, G., "Private Cost Containment", *New England Journal of Medicine*, Vol. 300, No. 23, pp. 1298–1305.

Howard, J. Keir, "The Prevention of Occupational Cancer: An ASTMS Policy Document – A Review", CIA Background Paper, 20 June 1980, Associations of Scientific Technical and Managerial Staffs. London, 1980. London, 1980.

Jones, R. Russell, "A problem which won't go away", *The Times*, 28 May 1980.

McLaren, Donald, letter to editor on mortality trends, *The Lancet*, 1 December 1979, p. 1183.

McMichael, John, letter to editor on cholesterol, *The Lancet*, 1 December 1979, pp. 1182–3.

Morris, J. N., "Are health services important to the people's health?", *British Medical Journal*, 19 January 1980, Vol. 280, pp. 167–8.

Morris, J. N., letter to editor, *The Lancet*, 3 November 1979, pp. 953–4.

"National survey on attitudes to smoking: minister's talks with tobacco industry still proceeding", *The Times*, 10 May 1980.

"Occupational cancer deaths 'on the decline' ", *The Times*, 4 July 1980.

Osman, Arthur, " 'Too few' women having ante-natal tests", *The Times*, 6 May 1980.

Todd, J. E., *Children's Dental Health in England and Wales, 1973*, Office of Population Censuses and Surveys, Social Survey Division, H.M.S.O., 1975.

Todd, J.E., and Walker, A.M., *Adult Dental Health, Volume 1, England and Wales 1968–1978*, Office of Population Censuses and Surveys, Social Survey Division, H.M.S.O., 1980.

Waldron, H.A., *The Medical Role in Environmental Health*, published for The Nuffield Provincial Hospitals Trust by the Oxford University Press, 1978.

Medical Education

Blum, Alan, "Who Shall Study Medicine in the 1980's?", *Journal of the American Medical Association*, 22–29 August 1980, Vol. 244, No. 8, pp. 779–80.

Chapman, Carleton, "On the Definition and Teaching of the Medical Ethic", *New England Journal of Medicine*, Vol. 301, No. 12, 20 September 1979, pp. 630–4.

"Cut med schools 13% and many residencies 20%, U.S. panel urges", *Medical World News*, 29 September 1980, pp. 10–12.

Ferriman, Annabel, "BMA call for limit on training new doctors", *The Times*, 12 April 1980.

Fordham, Christopher, "The *Bane Report* Revisited", *Journal of the American Medical Association*, 25 July 1980, Vol. 244, No. 4, pp. 354–7.

"Government Takes Steps to Avert Glut of Doctors", *New York Times*, 2 September 1980, p. C–1.

Nurse Training Act of 1975, Second Report to The Congress, 15 March 1979 (revised), U.S Department of Health, Education and Welfare, 1979.

Parkhouse, J., and McLaughlin, C., "Career preferences of doctors graduating in 1974", *British Medical Journal*, 2 (1976) 630.

Reproduction and Birth

Ayd, Frank, "Fetology: Medical and Ethical Implications of Intervention in the Prenatal Period", *Annals of The New York Academy of Sciences*, Vol. 169, 1970, pp. 376–81.

Black, Sir Douglas (Chairman), *Report by the Working Group on Screening for Neural Tube Defects*, D.H.S.S., July 1979.

Bodmer, W. F., and Cavalli-Sforza, L. L., *Genetics, Evolution and Man*, W. H. Freeman & Co., San Francisco, 1976.

Bowman, James E., "Ethical Issues in Genetic Screening", *New England Journal of Medicine*, Vol. 287, p. 205, 1972.

Dickens, Bernard M., *Abortion and the Law*, MacGibbon & Kee, 1966.

Duncombe, David C., *et al.*, "Ethical Issues in Genetic Screening", *New England Journal of Medicine*, Vol. 287, p. 204, 1972.

Gaylin, Hillard, "Genetic Screening: The Ethics of Knowing", *New England Journal of Medicine*, Vol. 286, pp. 1361–2, 1972.

Hestoff, Charles, and Rindfuss, Ronald, "Sex Preselection in the United States: Some Implications", *Science*, Vol. 184, 10 May 1974, pp. 633–6.

Lappé, Marc, "Choosing the Sex of Our Children", *The Hastings Center Report,* Vol. 4, No. 1, February 1974, pp. 1–4.

Lappé, Marc, *et al.,* "Ethical and Social Issues in Screenings for Genetic Disease", *New England Journal of Medicine,* Vol. 286, pp. 1129–32, 25 May 1972.

Lappé, Marc, "The Genetic Counselor: Responsible to Whom?", *The Hastings Center Report,* Vol. 1, No. 2, September 1971.

Lappé, Marc, "Risk-taking for the Unborn", *The Hastings Center Report,* Vol. 2, No. 1, February 1972, pp. 1–3.

" 'Live' Abortus Research Raises Hackles of Some, Hopes of Others", *Medical World News,* 5 October 1973, pp. 32, 33, 36.

Memoranda on the Abortion Act 1967 and the Abortion Regulations 1968, The Medical Defence Union, 1968.

Morison, Robert, "The Human Fetus as Useful Research Material", *The Hastings Center Report,* No. 4, 1973, pp. 8–10.

Murray, Robert F., "Problems Behind the Promise: Ethical Issues in Mass Genetic Screening", *The Hastings Center Report,* Vol. 2, No. 2, April 1972, pp. 10–13.

Ramsey, Paul, "Screening: An Ethicist's View", in Hilton, Bruce, *et al.* (eds), *Ethical Issues in Human Genetics,* Plenum Press, 1973.

Reilly, Philip, *Genetics, Law, and Social Policy,* Havard University Press, 1977.

Stenchever, Morton, "An Abuse of Prenatal Diagnosis", *Journal of the American Medical Association,* 24 July 1972, Vol. 221, No. 4, p. 408.

Shaw, Russell, *Abortion on Trial,* Robert Hale & Co., 1969.

Woolf, Jenny, "So hard to escape the maternity ward's conveyor belt", *The Times,* 10 July 1980.

Drugs

"Amphetamine Quotas and Medical Freedom", *The Hastings Center Report,* No. 12, 1973, pp. 8–10, Institute of Society, Ethics, and the Life Sciences.

Chowka, Peter, "The Organised Drugging of America", *The Ecologist,* Vol. 9, Nos 4/5, August 1979, pp. 155–60.

"Doctors urged to cut use of tranquillizers", *The Times,* 28 March 1980.

Duster, Troy, *The Legislation of Morality, Law, Drugs and Moral Judgment,* Collier Macmillan, 1970.

Ferriman, Annabel, "Better drug guidance demanded for GPs", *The Times,* 3 June 1980.

Grinspoon, Lester, and Singer, Susan, "Amphetamines in the Treatment of Hyperkinetic Children", *Harvard Educational Review,* Vol. 43, No. 4, November 1973, pp. 515–56.

Halberstam, Michael J., "Too Many Drugs?", reprinted from *Forum on Medicine*, Vol. 2, No. 3, March 1979, and Vol. 2, No. 4, April 1979, The American Enterprise Institute for Public Policy Research, Washington, D.C., 1979.

Klerman, Gerald, *et al.*, "Controlling Behavior Through Drugs", *The Hastings Center Studies*, Vol. 2, No. 1, January 1974, pp. 65–112.

O'Brien, R. Barry, "New version of old drugs help boost Health Service bill", *Daily Telegraph*, 29 November 1979.

O'Brien, R. Barry, "Wasted spending on brand-names increases health costs by £25m.", *Daily Telegraph*, 27 November 1979.

Reinhold, Robert, "U.S. Wins Agreement on Warning to Doctors on Use of Tranquilizers", *New York Times*, 11 July 1980.

Wardell, William (ed.), *Controlling the use of Therapeutic Drugs*, American Enterprise Institute Studies in Health Policy, Washington, D.C., 1978.

Wardell, William M., and Lasagna, Louis, *Regulation and Drug Development*, American Enterprise Institute for Public Policy Research, Washington, D.C., 1975.

Mental Illness

Berthoud, Roger, "Beyond the headlines – dedicated service to the mentally ill", *The Times*, 2 June 1980.

Breggin, Peter, "The Return of Lobotomy and Psychosurgery", *Quality of Health Care – Human Experimentation, 1973*, hearings before The Subcommittee on Health of the Committee on Labor and Public Welfare, United States Senate, Ninety-third Congress, First Session, on S.974, S.878, and S.J. Res. 71, 23 February and 6 March 1973, Part Z, pp. 755–77.

Clare, Anthony, *Psychiatry in Dissent*, Tavistock Publications, 1976.

Engelhardt, H. Tristam, and Spicker, Stuart F., *Mental Health: Philosophical Perspectives*, D. Reidel Publishing Company, Dordrecht, Holland, 1978.

Gaylin, Hillard, "On the Borders of Persuasion: A Psychoanalytic Look at Coercion", *Psychiatry*, Vol. 37, pp. 1–9, February 1974.

Gaylin, Hillard, "The Problem of Psychosurgery", manuscript, The Hastings Center Reading 905.

Hodges, Lucy, "Mental Health Act changes promised", *The Times*, 13 September 1980.

Hodges, Lucy. "Mental health patients deprived of many freedoms, pressure groups complain", *The Times*, 28 July 1980.

Mark, Vernon H., and Ervin, Frank R., *Violence and the Brain*, Harper & Row, New York, 1970.

Mark, Vernon, and Neville, Robert, "Brain Surgery in Aggressive Epileptics", *Journal of The American Medical Association*, Vol. 226, 1973, pp. 765–72.

"Mental patients' charter for UN", *The Times,* 16 June 1980.

Parry, Hugh, *et al.,* "National Patterns of Psychotherapeutic Drug Use", *Archives of General Psychiatry,* Vol. 28, June 1973, pp. 769–83.

"Physical Manipulation of The Brain", *The Hastings Center Report,* special supplement, May 1973.

Restak, Richard, *Premeditated Man,* Penguin, 1975.

Rosen, Ismond (ed.), *The Pathology and Treatment of Sexual Deviation,* Oxford University Press, 1964.

Skultans, Vieda, *Madness and Morals,* Routledge & Kegan Paul, 1975.

Szasz, Thomas, *The Myth of Psychotherapy,* Oxford University Press, 1979.

Szasz, Thomas, *Schizophrenia,* Oxford University Press, 1979.

Venables, H. D. S., *A Guide to the Law Affecting Mental Patients,* Butterworth, 1975.

Williams, Thomas A., and Johnson, James H., *Mental Health in the 21st Century,* D. C. Heath & Company, Lexington, Massachusetts, 1979.

Death and Dying

Brain Death, determination of: Correspondence, *British Medical Journal,* Vol. 281, 25 October 1980, pp. 910–11, 1139–41.

Capron, Alexander, and Kass, Leon, "A Statutory Definition of the Standards for Determining Human Death: An Appraisal and a Proposal", *University of Pennsylvania Law Review,* Vol. 121, November 1972, pp. 87–118.

"Declaration on Euthanasia", Catholic Information Services, *Briefing,* 27 June 1980, Vol. 10, No. 23.

"A Definition of Irreversible Coma", Report of the Ad Hoc Committee of The Harvard Medical School to Examine the Definition of Brain Death, *The Journal of The American Medical Association,* 5 August 1968, Vol. 205, pp. 337–40.

"Diagnosis of Brain Death", Statement issued by Conference of Medical Royal Colleges and their Faculties in the U.K., *British Medical Journal,* 1976, Vol. 2, pp. 1187–8.

Fries, James F., "Ageing, Natural Death, and The Compression of Morbidity", *New England Journal of Medicine,* 17 July 1980, pp. 130–5.

Jonas, Hans, "Against the Stream: Comments on the Definition and Redefinition of Death", *Philosophical Essays: From Ancient Creed to Technological Man,* Prentice-Hall, New Jersey, 1974, pp. 132–40.

Nichols, Peter, "Vatican says sick need not always be kept alive", *The Times,* 27 June 1980.

Pallis, C., and MacGillivray, B., "Brain Death and the EEG", letters to the editor, *The Lancet,* 15 November 1980, pp. 1085–6.

"Refinements in Criteria for the Determination of Death: An Appraisal",

182 *The Unmasking of Medicine*

Report by the Task Force on Death and Dying of the Institute of Society, Ethics and the Life Sciences, *Journal of the American Medical Association*, 3 July 1972, Vol. 221, No. 1, pp. 48–53.

Saunders, Cicely (ed.), *The Management of Terminal Disease,* The Management of Malignant Disease Series, Edward Arnold, 1978.

Veatch, Robert M., "Brain Death", *The Hastings Center Report*, No. 11, 1972, Institute of Society, Ethics and the Life Sciences, pp. 10–13.

Walsh, Michael J., Moffat, Ronald, Corbishley, Thomas, Harriot, John F. X., and Lakeland, Paul (eds), *The Quality of Death,* Templegate Publishers, Springfield, Illinois, 1975.

Alternative Medicine

Bresler, David E., *Free Yourself From Pain,* Simon and Schuster, New York, 1979.

Law, Donald, *A Guide to Alternative Medicine,* Turnstone Books, 1974.

Worthington, Leonard, "Unorthodox Healing and The Law", unpublished manuscript.

Consumerism

Cranston, Ross, "Consumers and the Law", Modern Law Series, Weidenfeld and Nicolson, 1978.

Nader, Ralph, *Unsafe at Any Speed,* Grossman, New York, 1965; adapted, Bantam Books, Toronto, 1973.

The Royal Commission on Legal Services, Cmnd. 7648, Final Report, October 1979.

Index

Aberdeen, University of
  survey of medical treatments 31
abortion
  and medical ethics 89, 91, 92
accidents
  and health care 52, 57, 62
  numbers of 65
  see also road accidents
accountability
  and technological innovation 152
active intervention
  and handicapped 82
advertising industry
  and alcohol consumption 66
  and cigarette smoking 63
  as anti-health force 61
alcohol
  abuse 4
  consumption and illness 52, 66, 67
American Psychiatric Association 1, 2

back pain
  cost to health services 62
Barnard, C. 36
Bevan, A. 46
Birmingham
  lawsuit against oil companies 118
  negligence case 134-5
Black, D. 58
Black Report on Inequalities in Health
  58, 59, 74
body
  functioning of 20-1
brain-stem death
  determination of 162-6
Brandt, K. 143
breast cancer 38
  and mass screening 148
breast-feeding
  campaign against 65
British Medical Association 96, 124,
  126
British United Provident Association
  health survey 41
bronchitis
  cost to health services 62
Bryce, J. 17

cancer
  and Laetrile controversy 39
  cases and GPs 33
  deaths in the United States 29
  of the lung 52, 63
  see also breast cancer
Carnegie Foundation 23
categorisation
  of patients 14-15, 111-114
  see also taxonomical categorisation
chemotherapy 149-50, 156
child health
  and preventive medicine 70-4
cholera 60
chronically ill 15
  and concept of illness 16
cigarette smoking
  and health 52, 62
  cost to health services 63-4
community care
  underdevelopment of 34, 55, 56
Community Health Councils 125, 126
community medicine
  decline in interest 56
community physicians 34, 56
competence
  and medical decision-making 79, 80,
  89
complaints procedure 126-7
congenital abnormalities
  cases and GPs 33
consultants
  choice of treatment 31
  distinction awards 36-7
consumerism 116-39
contraception
  and medical ethics 89, 91
coronary care 37
cost-benefit analysis
  and health care policy 145
court actions
  and improvement of health care 118-
  19
  and medical decisions 84-5
  see also litigation
Court Report on Child Health Services
  56-7

criminal law
  interrelationship with mental illness
    108-9
cure
  concept of 28-30
cryogenics 154

deaf people
  poor services for 72-3
death
  'chemical' 150
  code of practice 164-5
  definition 160, 161-4
  denial of 155, 158
  determination of 121, 164-5
  main causes of 52
  societal preoccupation with 15, 16,
    153-4
  see also perinatal mortality
Department of Employment
  and occupational health service 57
Department of Health & Social Security
  50, 121, 122
developing countries
  developments in health care 35
deviance
  and illness 11
diagnosis 16, 21
  and non-communication 87
  as problem-solving 29-31
diet
  and ill-health 52, 64-5, 68
disabled see handicap
disease
  concept of 18-19, 20, 21, 22, 30, 102
  elimination of 18-20
  identification 24-5, 31
distinction awards 36-7
doctor-patient relationship 88, 156
  and consumerism 130-1
  and litigation 132, 134
  and technological innovations 151
doctors
  and health education 62
  as agents of social system 12, 17, 48
  as scientists 22
  decision-making 76-98
  in industry 57
  planning numbers 43-4
  power of 2, 7-9, 89, 104
  roles 47-9
  self-regulation 124
  status 15

see also community physicians;
  consultants; general practitioners;
  hospital doctors
doctrine of informed consent 129-30
drug
  abuse 4-5
  costs 13, 36, 45
  induced coma 165
  production 23
  promotion 32, 45-6
  research 38-9
  side-effect 24
  see also tranquillisers
dying
  and ethical duty 156-60
  as an illness 15, 28-9, 154-5
  care of 155-6
  truth about 86
  see also death; terminally ill

economic restraint
  and improvement of health care 52
  effect on child health 73
  effects on health services 69
elderly see old people
Eli Lilly Co. 23
environmental health 68
equipment see technology
Erlich, P. 23
ethics
  and care of the dying 156-60
  and health priorities 49-50
  and medical decisions 78-98, 150-1
  and technological innovations 147-8,
    151-2
  and transplants 148-9
euthanasia
  voluntary 159
Exit 159

families
  and organ donation 149
family planning
  and medical ethics 90
  see also contraception
financial planning 53-4, 68-9, 145
  see also economic restraint; resource
    allocation
Flexner, A. 23
fluoride
  and reduction of tooth decay 73, 144
foetal screening
  and medical decisions 89, 95, 96

France
    maternity and child care services 70
fringe medicine 80

Gates, F. 47
General Medical Council 123, 138
general practitioners 13, 34
    and drugs promotions 45-6
    and health education 55
    and patient contact time 21
    post-graduate training 55
    types of consultation 33, 47-8
Genetic Manipulation Advisory Group
    122
gross domestic product
    and health care expenditure 43, 53

handicap 15, 16
    and concept of illness 14, 16
    and genetic counselling 89, 93
    and medical decisions 80-2, 93, 94
    neglect of sufferers 35, 42, 67-8
    see also spina bifida
health
    and mass screening 41
    and mental well-being 21
    as ability to work 9
    concept of 16-8
    definition of 17
    see also child health; mental health
health care
    improvements in 53-8
    in Soviet Union 32
    inequalities 58-9
    obstacles to 51-3
    see also National Health Service
health education 61-2
    and consumerism 117-18
    and lifestyles 53
    importance of GP 55
Health Education Council 61, 66
health education officers 62
Health Services Commissioner 125,
    127, 139
health visitors 61-2
heart disease 60
heart transplants 1, 36
    and health care resources 54, 122
Hoffman-La-Roche
    and Valium 48
homosexuality 1, 2
hospice movement 155

hospitals
    and concentration of resources 32-3,
        34-5, 54
    tasks 48-9
    see also mental hospitals; teaching
        hospitals
hospital doctors
    as an elite 33, 34
    roles 48-9

Illich, I. 13
illness
    and lifestyles 52-3
    and morality 4, 6, 8
    and social class 10-11, 14, 72-4
    as escape from responsibility 6, 12-13
    as possession 6, 18, 31
    as status 8-9, 40, 107, 110-11
    concept of 2-3, 6-7, 13-15, 24, 41-2,
        100-1
    definition 2, 18
    diagnosis 16
    see also disease; mental illness; specific
        illnesses
information
    about patient's condition 86-7
    dissemination and consumerism 117
    giving and ethics 96, 152
insurance
    doctors' 131, 137
    for medical care 131
    see also British United Provident
        Association
interferon 38-9
invalid 14
    and concept of illness 16

James, J. 50

Kennedy, E. 45
Kerr, J. 45
kidney dialysis 147
Koch, R. 22

labour economics 9-10, 14
Laetrile 39
language
    of medicine 1-2, 14
legislation
    and consumerism 125
    and health care 66-7
life expectancy 35, 53, 67
litigation 128-9, 133
Lorber, J. 93

mass-screening procedures 14, 41, 148
   see also foetal screening
Mather, C. 4
measles
   in Ecuador 22
   Oxfam vaccination programme 36
media
   and health education 62-3
medical decisions
   and ethics 78-98, 150-1
   definition 77
medical education 22-3, 27-8, 43
   and ethics 97
   postgraduate training for GPs 55
   see also teaching hospitals
medical officer of health *see* community
   physician
medical practice
   and consumerism 117-39
   and   technological   innovation
      36-9, 46, 140-4
   as political enterprise 2
   as problem-solving 29-30, 31, 32-3,
      44
   as a science 27-8
   audit of standards 124-5, 139
   codes 97-8, 121, 152-3
   problems of institutionalised frame-
      work 22
   standards 133
medical research 38-9
   and causes of illness 60
   and cigarette smoking 63
   and views of consumers 119-23
Mental Health Act 1959 110
mental hospitals
   admissions 110
   running costs
mental illness
   and biochemical malfunctioning 102
   and hospital care 48, 110
   as abnormality 105-7
   categorisation of patients 111-14
   incidence of 107
   language of 101, 110
   perpetuation of 14, 40
   problems of defining 99-105
Middle East
   growth of hospitals and equipment
      35
Miller, H. 28, 155
moral judgements
   and drug abuse 4-6

   and illness, 4, 6
   and mental illness 108-9
   by doctors 8
morphine addiction 4-5

Nader, R. 118
National Cancer Act 1971 29
National Child Development Study 74
National Enterprise Board
   and United Medical Enterprises 35
National Health Service
   expenditure on drugs 13, 36, 44-5
   expenditure on hospitals 32
   failure of 51-3
   reorganisation 55-6
   resource allocation 50
   workforce 27, 33
negligence 133-7, 138-9
   awards 134
   compensation for 131-2, 137-8
Nixon, R. 29
nurses 27, 33

occupational health service 34
   underdevelopment of 57, 65
old age
   and hospital care 48
   problems of 40, 67-8
ombudsman   *see*   Health   Services
   Commissioner
organ donation 148-9
Oxfam 36

parenting
   and medical decisions 90-1
patient
   as consumer 123
   as a person 21, 30
   categorisation 14-15, 111-14
   self-determination 133
   'social worth' 83, 95
patient participation groups
   in general practice 128
peer reviews 124
perinatal mortality 53
   and social class 58, 71-2
   in developing countries 35
   stillbirths 82
petroleum industry
   and pharmaceutical industry 23

pharmaceutical industry
  and general practitioners 45
  and medical education 22
  growth 23
  see also drugs
Pharmaceutical Society of Great Britain
  45
pharmacology 23, 24
poliomyelitis 38
  allocation of vaccine by lottery 150
political influences
  and health 17, 51, 52
  and medicine 2
possession
  and illness 6, 18, 31
poverty
  and educational achievement 74
  and illness 17, 40, 67-8
power
  and doctors 2, 7-9, 89
  and mental illness 100, 104, 110
pregnancy
  and social class 72
  and medical ethics 89
  as illness 40
  effects of cigarette smoking 63
  health care in France 70
  screening in 89, 95, 96, 121
prescriptions
  and drug addiction 5
  and drug promotion 45-6
  and financial savings 44-5
  for mood-changing drugs 13
pressure groups
  and health care improvements 118,
    128
preventive medicine
  and child health 70-4
  and health education 61-3
  and political action 61
  and resource allocation 17, 46, 58-9
  obstacles towards 63-70
  promotion of 49, 57-8
primary care 46
  and preventive medicine 55
professional audit 124

quality of life
  as criterion for medical decisions 81-
    2, 92, 94-5
Quinlan, K. 1
  court case 85

randomised controlled trials 124-5
recovery
  and concept of illness 14, 15
reductionism 30
resource allocation
  and health priorities 50, 54-5, 144
  and medical decisions 81
  concentration in hospital care 32-5,
    54
respirators
  and the dying patient 157-8
responsibility
  and illness 6, 12-13
  and mental illness 100
  of scientists 142-3
road accidents
  and drinking 66
  and health services 52, 55
  and speed limits 68-9
  and use of safety belts 65
  child deaths 73
Road Traffic Act 1967
  effects of 66
Rockefeller Foundation 23, 47
Royal College of General Practitioners
  study of general practice 33

St Thomas's Hospital Medical School
  mass-screening study 41
Salvarsan 23
Samaritans 114
Saunders, C. 155
school health service 34
  demoralisation of 56
Schweitzer, A. 36
science
  and medical education 27
  and modern medicine 26
  and responsibility 142-3
Senate Labour and Welfare Committee
  45
sickness certificates 10-11
Snow, J. 60
social class
  and ascription of illness 10-11, 14
  and child health 72-4
  and drug abuse 5
  and health 58-9
social conditions
  improvements and effect on health
    19
social problems
  and general practice, 11-12, 47-8

and illness 17, 67-8, 74
and old age 40
see also poverty
social security
and ill-health 67
social services
and resources allocation 68, 69
Soviet Union
hospitals and health care 32
specialisation
in hospital medicine 33-4
spina bifida
and antenatal screening 121
and medical decisionmaking 81
status
and being ill 8-9, 40, 107, 110-11
of doctors 15
Sweden
care of handicapped babies 82
Sydenham, T. 20
syphilis 23
Szasz, T. 100-1

taxation
and alcohol sales 69
and tobacco industry 64, 70
incentives and preventive health 69
taxonomical categorisation
of disease 21, 22, 31, 40
of mental illness 103, 110, 114
teaching hospitals 33, 34-5
technology
and medical ethics 96, 147-8, 151-2
and medical practice 36-9, 46, 140-4
in hospital care 54-5
terminally ill
and concept of illness 15, 16
and technology 37
care of 97
therapeutic privilege 87
tooth decay
cost to health services 62, 73
tranquillisers 11, 12, 13
over-prescribing 48
transplant surgery 98
and death 121
and kidney disease 147
and organ donation 148-9
and organ removal 148, 160-1
see also heart transplants

treatment
and the dying patient 156-8
as action against disease 31
tuberculosis 19, 22

Uganda
life expectancy 35
starvation problems 50
unemployment
and ill-health 67
United Medical Enterprises
sales of medical equipment 35
United States of America
cancer deaths 29
consumerism movement 118
court actions and medical profession 84-5
drug abuse 5
drugs promotions 45-6
ethics committees and medical research 122
GDP and health care 53
glut of doctors 43
Laetrile controversy 39
medical education 23
medical insurance 131-2
preoccupation with death 154
Professional Standards Review Organisations 124
screening for chemical suscepti-bility 41
Valium prescriptions 48

vaccination and immunization
against measles 36
against polio 38, 150
compensation for damage 138
loss of confidence in 72
value of 19
values
and ascription of illness 10-14
and decision-making 78, 146-7
and defining mental illness 108
and norm changes 4
and preventive medicine 64
and medical care 47, 51, 59, 145
and research 142-3
vitamin B *see* Laetrile

well-being *see* health
West Germany
  GDP and health care 53
women
  and child bearing 3–4
  and tranquillisers 11
  in social system 11–12
work

accidents and health services 52, 57,
  62
capacity and illness 9
satisfaction and longevity 67
World Health Organisation 17

Young, G. 61